LESSONS
FROM THE
COVID
WAR

AN INVESTIGATIVE REPORT

THE COVID CRISIS GROUP

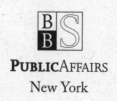

PUBLICAFFAIRS
New York

PublicAffairs
Hachette Book Group
1290 Avenue of the Americas, New York, NY 10104
www.publicaffairsbooks.com
@Public_Affairs
Printed in the United States of America
First Edition: April 2023

Published by PublicAffairs, an imprint of Perseus Books, LLC, a subsidiary of Hachette Book Group, Inc. The PublicAffairs name and logo is a trademark of the Hachette Book Group.

The Hachette Speakers Bureau provides a wide range of authors for speaking events. To find out more, go to www.hachettespeakersbureau.com or email HachetteSpeakers@hbgusa.com.

PublicAffairs books may be purchased in bulk for business, educational, or promotional use. For more information, please contact your local bookseller or the Hachette Book Group Special Markets Department at special.markets@hbgusa.com.

The publisher is not responsible for websites (or their content) that are not owned by the publisher.

Editorial production by Christine Marra, *Marra*thon Production Services.
www.marrathoneditorial.org
Print book interior design by Jane Raese
Set in 12.5-point Adobe Garamond

Library of Congress Cataloging-in-Publication Data has been applied for.

ISBNs: 978-1-5417038-0-3 (paperback), 978-1-5417038-1-0 (ebook)

LSC-C

Printing 1, 2023

CONTENTS

1

FROM TRAGEDY
TO POSSIBILITY

WE WERE SUPPOSED to lay the groundwork for a National Covid Commission. The Covid Crisis Group formed at the beginning of 2021, one year into the pandemic. We thought the U.S. government would soon create or facilitate a commission to study the biggest global crisis so far in the twenty-first century. It has not.

The thirty-four members of our group have done a lot of work on the Covid war, both as part of this group and in our day jobs. We held listening sessions with nearly three hundred people. We organized task forces. We mapped out agendas. We shared insights across our different backgrounds and did a substantial amount of research.[1]

We have learned a lot. With no commission in sight, we feel a duty to share, at the beginning of 2023, how we size up the Covid war.

A year into the crisis, we spoke with a doctor named Ashish Jha, who is now coordinating the government's Covid response. Back in 2021 he told us how, with the constant early mornings and late nights, he still couldn't process what he had been going through for more than a year. Being a medical doctor, naturally he had a diagnosis. He called it "reflection deficit disorder."

This short book is designed to alleviate the symptoms of reflection deficit disorder. It is a short course of treatment, available to all sufferers.

This disorder, this amnesia, can kill. We talked to a key figure in the crisis, one of those who helped originate the successful Operation Warp Speed that rushed vaccines to Americans, Peter Marks. Marks said it was stunning to him that there was so little understanding of the lessons from this war. Some experiences troubled him, Marks admitted. Sometimes he wished that, like one of those characters in the movie *Men in Black,* someone could administer a "neura-lyzer" and blank out his memories of certain meetings. But as Marks watched what was happening in the continuing Covid war, it seemed to him, at the end of 2022, as if the U.S. government and the country were "repeating the same mistakes" he remembered from the spring of 2020.

We do not promise a permanent cure for reflection deficit disorder. We cannot offer the kind of exhaustive investigative report that a Covid commission might have produced, interviewing layers of officialdom across the country and around the world, and piecing together thousands of key documentary records.

What we can offer is our sketch of the whole picture, our sense of how we think the pieces fit together. There are already many books and stories about this war. We step back and appraise the entire landscape, focusing on what we believe mattered most.

We have an advantage. Working together, we helped each other make sense of this overwhelming experience. Our take goes beyond some of the stock narratives. Our views don't fit neatly with partisan political arguments on either side in American politics. We believe this is a strength.

We wrote this book for our fellow citizens, experts and non-experts alike, who have already read hundreds if not thousands of articles about the pandemic as it happened. We will not spend much time just recapitulating what you likely already know.

We try to be more analytical, to zoom in on what mattered most. While being analytical, we have tried to write plainly. We are not writing the way we would write up our results for a scientific or medical journal. We think you, like us, want to get past the enormous jumble of information and make some sense of it all. What just happened to us, and why? How could we do better?

A GLOBAL WAR

We think it helps to see this crisis as a war—a global war. Some of us who work in healthcare don't like these sorts of warlike metaphors. Some of us do. Conceiving of this struggle as a "war" does help people think about how to organize collective action against a terrifying danger.

By the end of January 2020, the U.S. government should have started mobilizing to a war footing against a terrifying pandemic danger. It was not ready to do this. It did not start really trying to mobilize fully until about two months later, and even then in a haphazard way.

The world waged a war against an alien invader. In this case, the invader was not some giant from outer space. It was not an unknown threat. It was a viral microorganism, invisible to the naked eye. In all of human history, only during the last hundred years have humans even been able to see a virus. Rather than say "alien," scientists just say a new virus is "novel." When the invader is especially contagious and deadly, racing beyond some particular region, we call these invasions "pandemics."

Throughout human history, pandemics have been on the short list of the gravest threats to society and civilization. An outbreak of plague in the sixth century helped usher in what people recall as the "dark ages." Another such outbreak in the fourteenth century nearly destroyed large swaths of the populations in both Europe and Asia. Outbreaks of smallpox wrecked societies throughout the Western Hemisphere after the arrivals of Europeans. The great influenza virus pandemic of 1918–19 killed more people than the First World War.

Though it was perhaps no more than one-fourth as deadly per infection as the 1918–19 influenza virus, the COVID-19 pandemic was the most deadly and disruptive global pandemic since that one.[2]

The risk of these threats has sped up. The world has changed. In our extremely interconnected world, with its novel pressures on wildlife habitats, its interactions with livestock, its burgeoning experiments with synthetic biology, and the impact of climate change on biological risks, there is no particular reason to assume there will not be another such pandemic, relatively soon, in a matter of years, not centuries. This is why we must take a hard, searching self-inventory, right now, and face what we find.

COVID-19 is the name of a disease, Coronavirus Infectious Disease-2019. The disease is caused by a virus called

SARS-CoV-2. That is a way of saying Severe Acute Respiratory Syndrome, Coronavirus, Version 2. Version 1 broke out in southern China, between 2002 and 2004, and was at least twenty times more lethal per infection than our current Version 2.[3]

Fortunately for humanity, Version 1 spread more slowly than Version 2. Nor did Version 1 easily spread invisibly and asymptomatically. But this was a kind of biological luck. There is no law that guarantees a deadlier disease cannot also be extremely contagious. And there is no reason to assume the next one might not come soon. Or be deadlier.

Our story of the response to COVID-19 is about how American leaders and institutions handled a new kind of war. Given our own limitations, we will focus mainly on how Americans handled this war, but we keep an eye on what other countries did. And we keep in mind what other countries needed.

Imagine that you are a leader getting ready to wage such a war. You would face four basic challenges:

- *Prevent and warn.* Size up the danger, engage citizens, and track the enemy.

- *Contain the attack.* Keep the enemy out of the country or confine its spread.

- *Defend our communities.* Protect not only lives, but also our way of life, with proper healthcare and non-medical measures.

- *Fight back.* Develop and deploy medical countermeasures such as tests, medicines, and vaccines.

And it was a global war against a global invasion. All these things needed to be done rapidly and on a global scale.

THERE WERE HEROES.
THERE ARE LESSONS.

The world war against this invader, COVID-19, has not gone well. No country's performance is more disappointing than that of the United States.

America went into this war with unsurpassed scientific knowledge. Once at war, its politicians were willing to spend whatever it took. Thousands of people and organizations made heartrending, life-saving efforts. Yet our institutions did not meet the moment. They did not have adequate practical strategies or capabilities to prevent, to warn, to defend their communities, or fight back in a coordinated way, in the United States and globally.

The members of our group are angry. They are angry because they feel that good Americans, all over the country, were let down by ineffective institutions, a slow and uneven initial response, shoddy defenses, and inadequate leadership. We came away from many of our discussions consistently impressed with the ingenuity and dedication of people all over the country, and beyond. That is why so many of us are so frustrated. Americans improvised to fight this war, usually doing the best they could. They had to struggle with systems that made success hard and failure easy.

Yet those heroic improvisations—if we notice them— show us what might be possible. They reveal ingredients of a better system, a true national health security enterprise. At the state and local levels, governors and mayors began improvising citizen groups and "fusion cells" that, in real time, linked health departments, healthcare providers, emergency managers, business and community leaders. They shared daily updates on patient loads. Governors issued executive orders to force hospitals to coordinate how they handled surges and underserved towns.

At the federal level, the CDC (the Centers for Disease Control and Prevention) began experimenting with how to get better situation awareness, as the public system does in Israel, by finally starting to plug into healthcare data systems the way they do routinely in Britain. A new federal program, designed by little-known bureaucrats, Operation Warp Speed, showed new ways to power up extraordinary medical defenses on a revolutionary scale and fight back. The ideas are coming into view. The institutions now need to catch up.

There is no way to assess American performance without noticing the role of President Donald Trump. We will comment on that, where relevant. But during one of our group's many Zoom discussions, one of us just looked up and observed: "Trump was a comorbidity."[4]

Many Americans now understand that term. It represents a condition, a circumstance, that heightens risk of illness and death. But we also have to consider other factors too, so that enduring lessons can be learned.

Chapter by chapter, we will detail failures. But we also try to understand them. Most people did the best they could under the circumstances, often working frantically for long hours, week in and week out.

We will highlight some of their crisis-driven innovations, in America and beyond. This crisis is the occasion for a deep rethink of the way Americans organize and connect our haphazard system of healthcare, public health, practical policy-making, risk communication, medical countermeasures, and global defenses.

In a time of so much worry and disillusionment, the war has revealed new ways people around the world could help each other. New technologies also offer remarkable possibilities. As we reflect on this pandemic, arguments about whether to make the CDC director a Senate-confirmed position, or tinker at the margins of this or that program, seem like rearranging the deck chairs after the *Titanic* hits the iceberg.

THE AMERICAN TRAGEDY

The pandemic is tragic for all because of its toll on lives and livelihoods. It is tragic for America because no country went into the crisis with more scientific knowledge or spent more money, yet with such depressing results. And it is doubly tragic for America because the Covid war seemed to be a punishing reminder that, yet again, our governance, once regarded as the most competent in the world, was, well, not.

By late 2022, the Covid war had already likely caused about 20 million premature deaths around the world, with no end in sight. More than 1.2 million of these deaths were in the United States. About one-third were young or middle-age, a staggering toll even if no one above the age of sixty-five had died.[5]

We think at least 7 million Americans were hospitalized by Covid in the first two years of the pandemic. Many of the millions of survivors suffer lasting symptoms or disabilities from the disease. The pandemic made all of America's existing health inequities even worse: it hit hardest at the elderly, at rural communities, and at black, Hispanic, American Indian, Alaska Native, Native Hawaiian, and other Pacific Islanders.[6]

Since there are many problems with ascertaining who died from Covid, the most reliable estimates just look at how the number of total deaths compare with the number that would statistically be expected. This is a measure of "excess" mortality. We have relied upon excess mortality figures produced by the CDC, WHO, the network that monitors mortality in Europe (EuroMOMO), and the *Economist* to draw conclusions about comparative performance.[7]

For the United States, a sprawling country with over 330 million inhabitants, the fairest comparison is probably with the European countries and regions that are monitored in the European network. They constitute another sprawling community with over 368 million inhabitants. The Europeans have comparable though somewhat lower incomes. The most important demographic indicator of Covid vulnerability is age. In 2020, the median age of the EuroMOMO group was four years higher than that of the United States, so it helps to use age-adjusted comparisons.[8]

In 2020 and 2021, using common methods for the estimates and adjusting for age, the U.S. excess mortality rate was about 40 percent higher than the rate monitored among the Europeans. If the U.S. rate had been the same as that among the Europeans, the United States would have had 391,000 fewer deaths in those two years; the total differential in excess deaths by the end of 2022 probably approximates at least half a million. Then there are all the multiples of that in serious illness and other costs.[9]

Another kind of comparison, without these special adjustments, might just look, for instance, at the largest state in the United States with a median age above forty, which is Florida with a median age of about forty-two. Compare Florida to Spain, one of the warmer coastal countries in the European Union, with a median age of about forty-four. Spain performed about 50 percent better in saving its citizens from premature death than Florida did. If instead we compared Florida to Italy, a country with a still older population (median age of about forty-six), the difference shrinks. But Italy, with its much more elderly population, still performed about 30 percent better than Florida.

The other costs of the pandemic, in money spent, or disruption of commerce, or isolation and loneliness, or loss of schooling, are incalculable. Just the fiscal costs stretch our imagination. For instance, the Congressional Budget Office estimates that, between the first quarter of 2020 and the third quarter of 2021, the federal government deployed more than *$5 trillion* in fiscal policy responses to deal with the pandemic, including tax cuts or rebates. *That amount was more than a trillion dollars larger than the **entire** budget of the federal government, mandatory and discretionary, in fiscal year 2019.*[10]

A number that large is hard to grasp. A billion dollars is a lot of money. The lost economic output to the United States from the terrible 9/11 attacks was about $50 billion. Yet that amount is little more than a rounding error in comparison to the costs of the Covid war, about one percent of the $5 trillion that the federal government spent just through the third quarter of 2021. And that number is actual federal money spent. It does not include state and local spending.[11]

That number also does not include uncompensated costs in economic output, business failure, lost education, or unemployment. Economists David Cutler and Lawrence Summers, estimating the costs of lost lives and lost GDP in the United States, called Covid the "$16 trillion virus." That is an amount equivalent to nearly three-quarters of the entire American gross domestic product in 2020. And these U.S. numbers are, of course, just a fraction of the costs suffered and still being suffered by the rest of the world.[12]

Almost any calculation of return on investment would imply considering vastly more spending on health security, thinking in multiples of five or ten, compared to what the United States or other countries were spending in 2019. Writing about pandemic preparedness, economists use phrases like "spending billions to save trillions." This is not hyperbole. One group of economists that includes Susan Athey and the Nobel prize winner Michael Kremer has explained that, since the damages run in billions of dollars per day, even programs designed better to gain marginal advantages, that might shave just a month or two off the timeline of vaccine deployment, would still yield enormous benefits. Operation Warp Speed cost nearly $30 billion. It would be hard to find an expert to say that was too much. Instead, they wonder if the program should have spent much, much more.

Beyond all the disturbing statistics, one of the worst consequences was that Americans sensed their governance had let them down. It had let them down in performing the most fundamental task governments are expected to perform, to protect them in an emergency. Citizens know any community can face misfortune. Most accept that even good, dedicated officials can't do everything. But a mass crisis forces a lot of people to size up, according to their lights, how well they think their authorities faced the challenge, given the capabilities at hand.[13]

The United States of America faced the Covid invasion with more capabilities than any other country in the world. In October 2019, just before the pandemic surfaced, the Center for Health Security at Johns Hopkins, the Nuclear Threat Initiative, and the *Economist* published a landmark index of health security capabilities. Though no one received a perfect score, the authors gave the United States an 83.5, the highest score in the world. Spain and Germany both had scores of about 66. Italy earned a 56.[14]

Some people later mocked this index. But the authors worked hard to measure what they could, though they did not take full account of how little the United States spent on public health. It is hard to measure competence. It is hard, away from the front lines, to size up the human and institutional software that translates assets into effective performance. But it is also hard not to agree with Fareed Zakaria, who looked back on this index and commented that "by March 2020, these advantages seemed like a cruel joke." As

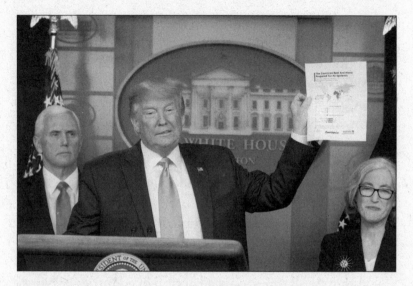

President Donald Trump at a White House briefing on February 26, 2020, flanked by Vice President Mike Pence and CDC Principal Deputy Director Anne Schuchat. Trump holds a copy of the Global Health Security Index while he explains the U.S. response to COVID-19. PHOTO CREDIT: TASOS KATOPODIS/GETTY IMAGES

Covid tore across the land, Zakaria wondered, "Was this the new face of American exceptionalism?"[15]

In the United States, it is sobering to compare the Covid pandemic of 2020–21 with the great influenza pandemic of 1918–19. In the world of 1918, knowledge of viruses and vaccines was in its infancy. Health and medical institutions were rudimentary. The doctors and nurses struggled, often valiantly, and were usually overwhelmed.

More than a hundred years later, in the world of 2020, the danger of a coming pandemic was predicted and publicized. Scientific knowledge was vastly more advanced.

Health and medical institutions were vastly more extensive. The money available was also vast; the U.S. Congress appropriated more than any country on earth. Millions of skilled Americans pitched in to help.[16]

Yet, for all their giant edifices, the net effect of the U.S. governance, public health, and medical institutions in 2020–21 seems all too comparable to the outcomes in 1918–19. This is true even as the developments of vaccines and treatments in 2020–21 were remarkable. And these health outcomes were attained at a stunning cost in shuttered businesses, lost jobs, demoralized citizens, disrupted education, and public debt.[17]

The whole world could have done better in handling this global war. At all times, only a handful of countries in North America, Europe, and Asia were able to lead. In principle, they could have built wartime coalitions with allied strategies, strategies from containment to product development to coordinated procurement on a global scale. Both America's Operation Warp Speed and the world's vaccine procurement entity, COVID-19 Vaccines Global Access or COVAX, were invented in the spring of 2020 in musings about what the world could do together. In practice, the lack of political will and preparation kept any real coalition effort from even getting to the runway.

Despite extraordinary efforts by countless committed individuals, the story of the Covid pandemic is the exact opposite of the story of the valorous but technologically feeble defense against the 1918–19 influenza pandemic. The Covid war is a story of how our wondrous scientific knowledge has run far, far ahead of the organized human ability to apply that knowledge in practice.

WHY ASK "HOW"?

When Zakaria asked, "Is this the new face of American exceptionalism?" his question was not rhetorical. His answer: "What matters is not the quantity of government but the quality."[18]

As we interviewed people throughout this crisis, the same question came up again and again: Is America still capable of solving big problems?

Caring about a problem is not enough. Public debates about policy are usually pleas to care about a problem. Then, if citizens care, they might commit themselves to do something about it. They might, for instance, spend a lot of their money and create some program to address the problem. But real policy work is less about the "should" and more about the "how."

In April 1947, the new American secretary of state, George Marshall, had just returned from a lengthy and worrying trip to Europe. Marshall had led the U.S. Army during the Second World War, the largest part of the largest enterprise ever undertaken by the U.S. government. His prestige was immense. He decided to broadcast a national radio address and brief the American people. He was supervising the development of an idea for European recovery that would later become known as the Marshall Plan.

Marshall did not announce that plan in his address. He just explained the situation. Drawing on some of that prestige he had earned, he asked his listeners to be patient with the details of what would be required. "Problems which bear directly on the future of our civilization cannot be disposed of by general talk or vague formulae—by what Lincoln called 'pernicious abstractions,'" Marshall warned. "They require concrete solutions for definite and extremely complicated questions."[19]

In October 2018, bestselling journalist Michael Lewis tried to call out the importance of "how." His book *The Fifth Risk* started from the premise that, in the twenty-first century, governments are risk managers. The federal government of the United States alone manages "the biggest portfolio of [catastrophic] risks ever managed by a single institution in the history of the world."[20]

Lewis did not focus on health security (though he later did that in his book on the Covid crisis, *The Premonition*, which features some members of our group). In *The Fifth Risk*, Lewis told compelling stories of little-known officials who do vital, unsung jobs.

One of Lewis's subjects was a man named Max Stier. Stier leads a nonprofit, Partnership for Public Service, that notices government success stories. Stier observed that "a surprising number of the people responsible for [these successes] were first-generation Americans who had come from places without well-functioning governments. . . . [P]eople who had never experienced a collapsed state were slow to appreciate a state that had not yet collapsed."[21]

Americans have more experience now. They now know what a collapsed government can feel like. In her memoir, former Covid task force coordinator Deborah Birx writes: "In April 2020, nearly everything came undone." Indeed, a number of state and local authorities from around the country told us that, during April and May of 2020, the federal government's executive role in the day-to-day management of the Covid crisis effectively ceased to exist.[22]

THREE CULTURES OF GOVERNANCE

The best emergency response Americans have ever made to a peacetime national emergency was during the Great Mississippi Flood of 1927, which killed people from Virginia to Oklahoma and displaced roughly 1 percent of the entire U.S. population. The secretary of commerce, Herbert Hoover, already known as "the Great Humanitarian" for his handling of relief operations for starving Europeans during and after World War I, took charge. Hoover's performance made him the most admired man in America and put him in the White House in the election of 1928.

Hoover used national policy and local execution. He set up competitions to procure relief supplies at a fair price. He cut deals with the railroads to reduce freight charges. He organized plans for scores of refugee camps that housed or fed more than half a million Americans. Local leaders, often from chapters of the American Red Cross headed by prominent men in the community, implemented the plans. President Calvin Coolidge put Hoover into the military chain of command so he could issue orders to soldiers and sailors, while also organizing a rescue fleet with hundreds of vessels. Little of the cost was actually absorbed by the federal government.[23]

We tell this story to highlight the difference between talk and action. One part of what leaders do is to "represent." They represent concerns and values. They stand for goals. Most mass politics therefore occurs in the realm of culture.

In a great emergency, the balance shifts away from the world of postures and positions and poses, from the practice of politics as performance art. That still matters—public communication in a crisis is vitally important. But the balance decisively shifts.

It shifts more to the world of producing results on the ground, through operations and action. Every big city mayor who has to handle snowstorms knows this. When the weather forecaster predicts the blizzard, it's too late to start putting in orders to buy snowplows.

In normal times, the U.S. government may issue a "strategy." Such documents have devolved into usually just being statements of goals and aspirations. That is not real strategy.

Real strategy is a notion of how someone plans concretely to connect ends with means. It is a theory of the "how." It is realized in blueprints of design, and by organizing, funding, training, and equipping many people to play their part in this choreography, people who sometimes must do very difficult things.

There are three main cultures in governance. One is a culture of programs and process. People get authority and money for a program. They administer processes. Many programs are controlled more by congressional committees than by their nominal agency heads. The programs are created to dispense money and they do that, following the given process.

Another is a culture of research and investigation, sometimes to offer advice or inform regulation. It is the dominant culture of high science, the realm of basic research and some ethical reflection. Its strengths were apparent in this crisis in, for example, the understanding of molecular biology and the NIH's support for messenger RNA technology. The CDC nurtures cadres of disease detectives. It is a culture that can become insular, if the researchers mainly just judge each other, and judge only by their own cultural standards for methods, insight, and value.

A third is a culture of operations, to do things, to produce results in the field. It is a culture that can be resilient and adaptable, since the operators have to adjust to the real conditions they encounter in the field. It too can become insular and clannish in other ways. It is the dominant culture in most private firms, especially those that make products or deliver services. It is the dominant culture in a large part of the governance most Americans actually interact with every day, little of which is in the federal government.

The challenge in the Covid war, as in any great emergency, is to meld all these cultures in practice. It is very difficult to do this. What the Covid war exposed, what every recent crisis has exposed—even in Iraq and Afghanistan—is the erosion of operational capabilities in much of American civilian governance. The giveaway is how often governments and agencies had to hire management consultancies— McKinsey, the Boston Consulting Group, Bain & Co., and a number of others—to perform basic operational tasks.

These firms used to be thought of as outsiders that would occasionally be called in to assess the usual operators. What was telling in the Covid war, as in other wars, was how often such firms were asked to do the work itself, to staff leading officials and organize the management of the crisis. It is one thing to hire contractors to do specific work. It is another to outsource much of the policy design work itself. That is the point when government starts losing the know-how of governance.

The test of war or a great emergency puts a much greater emphasis on operational readiness and action. In the chapters that follow, we urge readers to notice the connections between the cultures of programs/processes, of research/investigation, and the people and organizations—private and public—who might have to conduct large operations.

In an emergency, either governments already have the trained people and equipment they will need, or they don't. If they don't, they can either give up or they can try to go get what they need from the private sector. This challenge of how to harness the private sector in an emergency would come up in a dozen ways during the Covid war.

The Covid war revealed profound gaps between officials who regarded the private sector from a detached, often regulatory, distance and those who, anticipating what they might need, wished to proactively mix it up and manage the required public-private partnerships. The irony is that the hands-off approach did not evade reliance on private firms. It just dealt with that reliance in the worst possible ways.

THE "SOFTWARE" OF POLICY COMPETENCE

Policy work, like any engineering that applies knowledge to practical problem-solving, is painstaking. Most people notice some of the "hardware" of policy: the resources, tools, and broad structures that frame the possibilities for useful work. That is important.

Less noticed is the "software" of how people actually do the substantive public problem-solving within these constraints. Such software overlaps with the formal structures of government, but it is really a different subject. These are the routines for the way the operational work is done: the methods people use to size up problems, design actions, record and reflect on what they are doing, and implement actions in the field. As any software developer can attest, such choreography can be a rigorous craft.

Especially in the middle of the twentieth century, America and its officials had once been famous all over the world for the quality of their public problem-solving. The world regarded us as the enterprising, imaginative problem-solvers, who could seem to do almost anything, in war or peace, with a practical, can-do spirit. American accomplishments ranged from D-Day to building atomic bombs to feeding millions amid the ruins of Europe and Asia to mounting Marshall Plans and Berlin Airlifts. We even helped the world join together to eradicate smallpox. Any close study of these efforts reveals superior construction of large-scale, multi-instrument policy packages, including frequent adjustments.

The organizational cultures of this era, which were closely related to the engineering-oriented business culture that reached its height in mid-twentieth-century America, were passed along mainly through imitation and apprenticeship. All this slowly faded later in the century. Official habits, routines for staff work, and professional cultures have changed a lot during the last fifty years. The software of public problem-solving has deteriorated. The reasons do not principally lie with the rise or fall of polarization in American politics. Those quarrels can be corrosive, but they are not new.

Successful problem-solving cultures had not come out of academia and they had not migrated back to academia.

Little had been done to preserve or teach the older skills. Unlike the methods taught for engineering, the software of policy staff work is rarely recognized or studied. It is not adequately taught. There is no canon with norms of professional practice. American policymaking has become less about deliberate engineering and more about improvised guesswork and bureaucratized habits.

Even before the Covid war, it seemed fair to judge that this earlier American reputation for practical public problem-solving had faded, especially after the wars in Iraq and Afghanistan. This pandemic crisis is so encompassing, has touched so many communities, that, as we understand it better, surely a teachable moment has arrived.

What follows is our take on what happened, how, and why.

LEARNING LESSONS

COVID-19 kills quietly. It does not kill with the violence of war or the shock of seeing young people collapse and die on the street, gushing out their lifeblood, as happened sometimes during the 1918–19 influenza pandemic. Covid usually kills out of public view. Most of the private healthcare system was able to muddle through Covid, on the backs of heroic healthcare workers and aided by an enormous government bailout.

Much of the obsolescent public health infrastructure was overrun. Public and rural hospital systems as well as many nursing homes were ravaged. But the biopharma industry and some portions of the healthcare system, especially in metro centers, did well out of the crisis. We are not surprised. After all, the American system is not designed to fight a global war against an alien invader. It is designed to provide healthcare. And the war sure generated a demand for that.

Though some people are trying, there is not yet any great push to fundamentally overhaul our public health or healthcare system, or to envision a better national health security enterprise. We find this alarming. The statistics may seem numbingly familiar—more than one million premature deaths, more millions in the hospital, more millions suffering from Long Covid, a quarter of a million children who have lost parents or other caregivers and are Covid orphans, closed schools and businesses, and the "distancing" of Americans from each other in so many ways, including the places where they pray, serve, and engage. Hardly any American has not been touched by this catastrophe.[24]

No large interest groups have emerged to press for change, except some tireless efforts by some associations and survivors (often stricken by Long Covid) and the families of some victims. Long Covid itself remains poorly understood. The victims include disproportionate numbers of the young and previously healthy.[25]

As Long Covid victims try to cope, they advocate for care and research on their illness. When we listened to representatives from four groups of Long Covid sufferers, one wearily said: "I just want to add that the vast majority of this work has been done by volunteers, many if not most of whom are still sick, and some of us, like myself, still trying to balance paid work as well."

The policy agendas of both major American political parties appear mostly undisturbed by this pandemic. There is no momentum to fix the system. Although several public health experts warned us about the usual cycle of "panic and neglect," it still is astonishing to watch that cycle repeat once again.

The Covid war revealed a collective national incompetence in governance. The leaders of the United States could not apply their country's vast assets effectively enough in practice. Trust and confidence in government—already low—further eroded. The most successful national program to wage the war to produce and distribute vaccines, Operation Warp Speed, ended up having to be run substantially by the Department of Defense.

Lessons already abound, as the pandemic continues to evolve, marked by the enormity of the delayed outbreak in China during the winter of 2022–23.

To learn those lessons, more than two years ago a group of foundations sponsored a substantial effort to prepare a national Covid commission. We provide more details about this at the back of the book, in the section "About the Covid Crisis Group." The foundations and the Covid Collaborative recruited Philip Zelikow to lead this planning group, since he had helped lead other bipartisan and nonpartisan examinations, including the 9/11 Commission.

The United States government has decided not to create such a commission. A bipartisan bill to establish such a commission passed out of committee in the Senate but never made it to the floor and died with the end of the 117th Congress.

The members of our group were disappointed, but not surprised. We saw that an effective commission would be unlikely in the current political environment. Each side already has its talking points about blame.[26]

One common denominator stands out to us that spans the political spectrum. Leaders have drifted into treating this pandemic as if it were an unavoidable natural catastrophe.

The American people know a lot about how the pandemic has affected their lives. They do not have a very good understanding of what happened. They do not see any evident agenda for change.

John Kingdon, a political scientist who wrote about how public agendas emerge, once explained that the difference between a "condition" and a "problem" lies in whether people think they can do something about it.[27]

In the absence of a clear picture, in the absence of constructive ideas for change, people become fatalistic. Their leaders are treating the pandemic as if it were an inescapable tragedy. It is as if a hundred years ago, accepting that life brings fires and floods, it never occurred to anyone that there could be such a thing as building codes or levees.

Confronting bad governance, fatalistic apathy would be un-American. And it dishonors the memory of what and who we have lost—and are still losing.

The most important lessons are not about structures and org charts. Memory of the 9/11 Commission's work is now receding into the past. That best-selling report led to some structural fixes, like the little-known National Counterterrorism Center, but its main impact back in the early 2000s was not bureaucratic. Its main value came from sharing understanding about what happened, what mattered, and what to do.

The United States met the 21st century pandemic emergency with structures mainly built for 19th century problems. Modernizing those structures turns out to be more about updating the software of governance than about disruptively rebuilding the nationwide hardware of federalism.

The main legislative response to the pandemic, enacted in December 2022, tweaked authorities and added some program funds. Congress added a new White House office for pandemic preparedness and policy response. That White House office may yet be put to good use, but it was an office that the Biden administration had not sought, and it comes without operational authority or budget power. Such organizational fixes may just compound crisis management confusion.

Some strategies have been announced, including by the Biden administration. But these "strategies" tend to be lists of goals, not road maps for accomplishing them.

Had these changes been in place in 2019, they might not have altered the outcomes very much, if at all. There will be other disease outbreaks, other emergencies. Citizens therefore need to understand this one, this Covid war.

Noticing the faltering political momentum, the void where there should be an agenda for change, our group decided to speak out.

2

ORIGINS, PREVENTION, AND WARNING

I F THE OUTBREAK had been prevented or contained in Asia when it surfaced in late 2019, there would have been no war at all. Perhaps there would just have been a faraway skirmish, known to or studied by experts, as people study the coronavirus outbreak that emerged in and near the Arabian Peninsula during 2012 called MERS (Middle East Respiratory Syndrome).

Below we sum up our view of the controversy about the origins of COVID-19. It is necessarily preliminary. There is not enough evidence available from inside of China to come down hard on any theory of the origins of the virus. Some more information may emerge from investigations into sources of evidence outside of China.

We believe strongly though that, regardless of how the origins controversy comes out, what is already known drives two great agendas for the future. First, we believe governments must improve their intelligence about what is going on—their situation awareness. The past system relied on national governments like China to provide timely reporting of what was happening. That system decisively failed. We need to envision an alternative.

In a war, intelligence is vital. It is vital at every stage, from prevention to warning to ongoing assessment of the danger and how the war is going. If the term "intelligence" seems out of place in a discussion of pandemics, then just think of it as a problem of situation awareness.

The primary task of any security system is to prevent or warn of an impending attack. The better methods for doing this formulate scenarios for how the greatest dangers might arise. Then they analyze how such developments might be detected. They put in place the means to do that detecting and validate how well that works in the real world. Then they figure out what to do when alarm bells start ringing.

Second, we suggest a large, difficult multinational effort to regulate the most risky research. That includes biosafety, biosecurity, and dual use research of concern.

THE ORIGINS ISSUE

Deadly pathogens arise in the natural world and humans encounter novel ones as they interact with the animal world. What is new in our history is that humans can also now engineer deadly pathogens in a lab, either *de novo*—from scratch—or by manipulation.

A coronavirus caused the severe acute respiratory syndrome (SARS) epidemic of 2002–04. That coronavirus, formally known as SARS-CoV-1, is thought to have originated naturally among bat populations in remote forests and caves in southeast Asia. Such bats and viruses have been found in southern China, northern Laos, northern Thailand, Cambodia, and Myanmar.[1]

But the first known spillover of this virus to humans, leading to the first SARS epidemic, appears to have taken place some distance away from those bat habitats, in the Guangdong province of China. In that epidemic, scientists hypothesized that the bats had passed the virus to some intermediary animal, like civets. The civets might then have been transported to wildlife markets in distant cities. In some farms raising wild animals for food, Chinese scientists found antibodies to that first SARS virus, which meant there might have been some circulation of that virus in those wildlife farms. At first, fruit bats were the prime suspects as the original source of the virus. Zhengli Shi, a program head at the Wuhan Institute of Virology, helped zero in on horseshoe bats.

In 2012, six miners in southern China's Yunnan province, working not far from the borders with Laos and Vietnam, presented with an unusual illness. Three of them died. Some medical practitioners believed the miners had caught a SARS-like virus. Following up, Chinese scientists from Wuhan discovered many SARS-like viruses among horseshoe bats from the same mine in Yunnan province where these miners had spent time immediately before they got sick, as well as among bats across southern China. Although related, none of the viruses found so far in this region or elsewhere are the immediate ancestors of the novel coronavirus, SARS-CoV-2, that has caused COVID-19.[2]

In that 2012 incident, the miners may have caught the disease directly from the bat feces (guano) in caves. After their years of post-SARS work to find suspect coronaviruses, Wuhan-based scientists collected samples of blood, feces, and other samples from those bats and took them back to Wuhan for study.

Wuhan is the capital city of Hubei province. It is a city of 11 million people in central China. It is hundreds of miles away from the places where most of the related bat-borne viruses have been found.

Since the COVID-19 pandemic first surfaced on a mass scale in Wuhan, there are two main hypotheses, or theories, about how it got to Wuhan and how it crossed over to humans.

The first theory is that humans transported wild animals carrying the virus to Wuhan.

This "spillover" theory is plausible. It is consistent with generally accepted theories about how the first SARS epidemic began in southern China. It is also consistent with theories about the emergence of Middle Eastern Respiratory Syndrome (MERS), which apparently jumped from bats to camels to humans in Saudi Arabia and was first identified in humans in 2012. Wild animals can clearly be carriers of coronaviruses. These hosts amplify transmission of these viruses and facilitate spillover to humans. And, importantly, in 2019 there were multiple wildlife markets in Wuhan stocking, slaughtering, and selling relevant animals.[3]

Since the 1980s, China had built up wildlife farming into a major industry. After research suggested that such farming might have produced the first SARS outbreak, the Chinese government banned wild game markets. Worried about

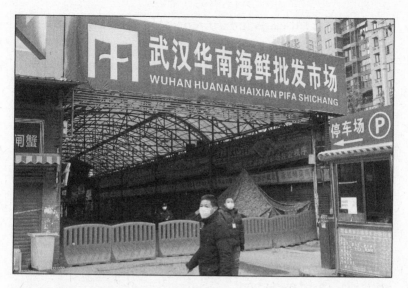

The Huanan Seafood Wholesale Market, in Wuhan, China, on January 17, 2020. An unusual proportion of the early reported cases of COVID-19 in China were clustered near this market, and it is at the center of debates about the origins of the virus. The market was closed by Chinese authorities on January 1, 2020. PHOTO CREDIT: KYODO NEWS VIA GETTY IMAGES

rural poverty in the three regions that bred such animals for affluent city-dwellers, these restrictions were soon lifted and the industry roared back.[4]

An unusual proportion of the early reported cases of COVID-19 seem to have clustered near one of those markets, the Huanan Seafood Wholesale Market, which sold live animals as well as seafood. (This market is a thirty-minute ride from the Wuhan Institute of Virology and quite close to Wuhan's Center for Disease Control.) This finding does suggest the possible importance of the wildlife market, *if* those reported cases indeed reflect the true distribution of early cases.[5]

However, the location of the cases at the very outset of the pandemic is uncertain. As the first major Chinese publication about the virus explained (on January 24, 2020), the clinical appearance of the early patients had "confounded early detection of infected cases, especially against a background of ongoing influenza and circulation of other respiratory viruses." In other words, the earliest cases of SARS-CoV-2 infection may have not been identified at the time or subsequently. And, because early Chinese investigators were suspicious about the Huanan market, they may have oversampled early cases there and undersampled potential cases elsewhere.[6]

Genomic analysis of samples from early cases gives another clue. It suggests the possibility that there were two early lineages of the viruses, both circulating at the same time among humans in November or December 2019. Patients infected with both lineages were associated with the Huanan market, and environmental samples taken from the market matched one of the lineages. These observations reinforce speculation that the pandemic might have originated with at least two separate spillover events.[7]

The multiple early lineages of the virus imply that there was more than one path of genetic mutation in hosts that crossed over to humans. As we will explain later, this could be consistent with the second leading theory concerning the research process, but it is more plausible as a product of crossover from different infected animals. The potential emergence of COVID-19 across multiple wildlife markets would mirror evidence that the first SARS outbreak might have come about in this way, one of several arguments made in an influential summary by a research group headed by Edward Holmes.[8]

The two lineages identified in some early cases of COVID-19 are distinguished from each other by different compositions of molecules (nucleotides) at just two of the roughly thirty thousand positions in the SARS-CoV-2 genome. The nucleotides at all other positions are identical. A variance of two positions is extraordinarily close and suggests little difference in evolutionary time between the two samples. It is the kind of difference that typically arises after several weeks of transmission among humans. There are some technical issues, including questions about the theoretical modeling, but the main issue is not whether there were independent lineages. It is more about when they became independent—the dates and locations of early cases.

The root of the problem of figuring out whether there were one, or two, introductions of the virus into humans is, again, that the dates and places of the earliest cases of COVID-19 have not been independently determined. We are not confident that anyone has identified "patient zero" in China. The Chinese authorities have not shared access to the primary biosurveillance data and samples about claimed early cases or the related records about their provenance.

One of us, Nicholas Christakis, believes it is possible to infer a possible timing for patient zero by looking at data from genetic mutation rates in early strains of the virus or the movements of large numbers of people and the timing of when the pandemic first surfaced in parts of China. Analyzing such data, in an early paper published in *Nature*, his research group estimated that the first people infected in

Wuhan might have left that city in late October or early November 2019 and could have been infected in early October.[9]

In 2022, in briefings for the World Health Organization, the official Chinese position was that they could not find a single sample of SARS-CoV-2 in any of the tens of thousands of animals they have tested in China, including from breeding sites for wildlife markets. They said that there were no such samples in any of the eighteen species of animals tested from the former Huanan wildlife market in Wuhan. Environmental samples from that market did have SARS-CoV-2, but all those samples could be linked to prior human infections.

The Chinese position, then, is that there is no hard evidence that the virus originated in China at all. "Anywhere But Here" was the title of an August 2022 article in *Science* summarizing recent Chinese papers. The Chinese government has stonewalled all independent research inside China that might delve further into this mystery.[10]

The second theory is that humans transported their collected virus samples back to a lab in Wuhan and that the virus crossed over to humans in some part of the research process, from collection to experimentation.

This "research process" or "lab leak" theory is also plausible. Scientists and their technical staff did collect and transport thousands of specimens from bats to Wuhan. These labs did have research programs to explore the possibility of bat-associated coronaviruses infecting humans.

Years before the emergence of SARS-CoV-2, scientists had noted the similarity of bat-associated coronaviruses to both MERS and SARS-CoV-1. They therefore knew bat-associated coronaviruses might be quite dangerous, that they had the potential for interspecies transmission to other animals and to humans. These scientists had urged enhanced surveillance that might detect another spillover event.

The research process theory has two main hypotheses. One is that a natural virus could have infected a human while collecting field samples in southern China, and this person traveled back to Wuhan before infecting others. In a related scenario, a lab worker might have infected themselves or others while trying to grow viruses from these samples in Wuhan. The last known human infections from the original SARS virus (the one in the 2002–03 outbreak) occurred because of lab accidents in Singapore, Taiwan, and China.[11]

The second hypothesis is that laboratory staff used modern genetic engineering tools capable of making a bat coronavirus more transmissible among humans and such experiments may have led to the creation of SARS-CoV-2. Such work might try to learn about patterns of mutation in the most dangerous viruses. It was the Wuhan Institute of Virology's general efforts to identify dangerous viruses that led a number of U.S. government agencies (USAID, NIH, Department of Defense) to support biological research in Wuhan. There is no firm evidence that such work, whether supported by Chinese or U.S. funders, did in fact create SARS-CoV-2. Yet we have limited information about the overall work being done in Wuhan or about the samples and viruses that were collected there.

For a number of years, scientists have conducted research to discover which viruses might have pandemic potential. They induce changes in the virus, a "gain of function," to discover pathogens with pandemic potential. For more than a decade, some scientists have been worried that a gain-of-function experiment might create an exceptionally dangerous novel virus. The U.S. government created the National Science Advisory Board for Biosecurity (NSABB) to reduce risk from "gain-of-function research of concern." The NSABB proposed guidelines. Studies that would make a virus more transmissible or virulent would require special review. In 2017, the outgoing Obama White House told agencies to develop such a framework. HHS complied that year; other agencies did not. In December 2022, Congress enacted a law requiring such reviews across the government.[12]

Because Chinese laboratories collected many specimens of bat-associated coronaviruses for SARS-related study, some of which share more than 95 percent sequence identity with SARS-CoV-2, some experts have expressed concern that one of these labs may have conducted experiments that could have inadvertently created more transmissible strains of the virus. Chinese investigators deny that their research was risky. They deny that their work created SARS-CoV-2.[13]

If a SARS-related virus that could infect humans was either brought into a lab in the process of collecting field samples or created through genetic manipulations, such a virus would still need to escape from the lab to infect the general population. There are three ways something like this could occur.

First, someone could have intentionally removed a dangerous virus, perhaps to use in a criminal release. Such an event apparently occurred in the October 2001 attacks in the United States that used anthrax—attacks which the U.S. Department of Justice eventually (in 2008) attributed to an anthrax scientist who took his own life shortly before charges were brought and a jury could weigh the evidence. We think this scenario is the least likely. No one has plausibly suggested that any pathogens were deliberately released from a lab working on coronaviruses. No perpetrator has claimed responsibility. But protecting against such dangers is one of the purposes of biosecurity regimes.[14]

Second, if a SARS-related virus transmissible to humans came into a lab, and especially if it was propagated in cell culture or laboratory animals, an investigator could have become infected through a lab accident—post-spill inhalation, or some other exposure. Investigators working on coronaviruses in Wuhan reported that they identified no lab-acquired infections among their colleagues. But the methods and primary data to support these reports have not been shared. Moreover, investigators may not have been focused on asymptomatic transmission at this early stage of the pandemic. Perhaps such cases were overlooked.

Third, the mechanical safeguards put in place to ensure that the lab itself was operating safely may have failed. Bio labs typically use four levels of biocontainment. Biosafety Level 2 (BSL2) uses routine biosafety measures such as limited access, biosafety cabinets when handling pathogens, no eating or smoking in the lab, and other elementary precautions. BSL2 labs are common around the world.

BSL3 labs have all the BSL2 safety measures and add special protective equipment to guard against aerosol exposure, directed airflow to maintain negative air pressure in the lab, and may add HEPA filtering of exhaust air. BSL3 labs are used in many government, academic, and industrial research facilities around the world.

BSL4 labs represent the highest level of biocontainment. They have many precautions built into their design to protect the people working there, the surrounding community, and the environment. They are very complex facilities. They are very expensive to build and costly to maintain. They require constant skilled engineering support. At present over fifty BSL4 labs are known to exist around the world. One began operating at the Wuhan Institute of Virology in 2017.[15]

According to Chinese investigators, earlier work with bat-associated coronaviruses in China was being conducted in BSL2 facilities, with some limited animal work done at the BSL3 level. BSL2 protocols are usually insufficient to protect against viruses transmissible as aerosols, such as SARS-CoV-2.

In addition to the absence of reports of a breach or of any lab-acquired infections among the coronavirus researchers, the press has reported that the Chinese armed forces have conducted their own thorough investigation of the Wuhan facilities. To a degree outsiders do not yet understand well, the Chinese armed forces were supporting research at the Wuhan Institute of Virology. Then again, so were agencies of the U.S. government that were hoping to learn how to prevent pandemics.[16]

Straightforward examination of Wuhan staff for evidence of laboratory-acquired infection or leaks in containment during the collection or research process could help outsiders understand whether the lab or its collection processes were a possible source of the pandemic. Our point is that such examinations were almost certainly done during the Chinese government's own investigations. But the results of those investigations have not yet been shared.

We also have to point out that the scientists at the Wuhan Institute of Virology work in a high-pressure political environment. In 2018 and 2019, leading Chinese scientists and public health experts had openly voiced concern about the limitations of their high-level biocontainment infrastructure, including problems with safety policies, education, and staff experience. Yet Chinese scientists also had to face significant pressure to compete with and overtake American and European scientific capabilities, pressure coming from the highest levels of the Chinese government. Chinese scientists were being pushed to show achievement "now." Such pressures can create a more risky environment for doing high-containment virology work.

We have spoken with leading scientists associated with both of the major theories for how the virus got to Wuhan— either due to animal-to-human spillover or via the research process.

Both theories remain plausible. As we said at the beginning of the chapter, more evidence about the origins of COVID-19 might emerge from investigations into sources outside of China. At present, we just do not think there is enough evidence available, yet, to come down hard either way.

The origins controversy is important in its own right, of course. But from the point of view of intelligence or situation awareness, and learning lessons, *both theories drive toward common, urgent insights for action.* Even if the first theory turns out to be correct, it is not very hard to come up with a scenario in which the second theory could have caused the pandemic. And vice versa. So any lessons have to be valuable either way.

IMPROVING SITUATION AWARENESS

Many kinds of human activity can produce threats to biological security. Some involve activities that cause climate change or the invasion of wildlife habitats; some involve large-scale farming and handling of poultry and livestock.

The Covid war points up two big strategies for this kind of common work. The first is transnational biomedical surveillance. "Surveillance," like "intelligence," sounds surreptitious. With open communications and clarity, and strong national systems that report to a global platform, it need not be.

This is not a utopian, unworldly suggestion. We spoke with Nancy Cox, a long-serving veteran of both the CDC and the WHO, with extensive field experience in China. Few did more to build up the Global Influenza Surveillance and Response System (GISRS). It is an interesting model, one that involves national governments, the WHO, and the UN's Food and Agriculture Organization.

"GISRS is credited," she reminded us, "with being the most fully developed global pathogen detection and identification system in existence," and she had not seen that claim credibly disputed. If adequately supported, it had the potential, she thought, to be "a global sentinel network for detecting and identifying new viral respiratory pandemic threats."

In an earlier time, Chinese efforts grew to become a bulwark of this system. Indeed, a number of Americans, including some members of our group, look back with great respect on decades of productive work on many subjects with highly skilled Chinese medical practitioners and virus researchers.

The world can no longer rely on governments in closed societies to provide voluntary, timely national reporting of an outbreak. Capable governments in more open societies must develop other ways to provide necessary biomedical surveillance.

At least four U.S. government agencies have or are creating centers to manage the biological intelligence challenge. All will have to do better than they did during the winter of 2019–20. Other countries are also creating new capabilities, as is the World Health Organization.

Surveillance to detect the introduction of an infection and identify possible cases can monitor "pre-healthcare" data streams, such as absenteeism from work or relevant internet search queries. Such surveillance can also be biomedical, looking at specimens that have been collected from patients, "syndromic" surveillance (which some hospitals do now), or sentinel and research efforts. Though it later turned out that Covid had already arrived, the first confirmation of a Covid case in the United States was detected because of the Seattle Flu Study, on the lookout for possible flu cases, despite being initially hindered by stringent Covid testing regulations.[17]

Some advocates seek to prevent a deadly biological invasion by protecting remote animal habitats. They hope to discourage or regulate dangerous new human-animal interactions. This is part of a "One Health" approach, treating the health of people, animals, plants, and their shared environment as a common, interactive ecology.

Policymakers have found it hard to turn this goal into practical programs that can actually be implemented where the dangers are greatest. But, at the end of February 2020, China did ban all trade and consumption of wildlife for food and began closing down this industry (again), compensating some breeders and farmers.[18]

Some have proposed conducting more thorough surveillance of animal populations to detect, collect, and study other potentially dangerous viruses. That was the kind of research program that animated the collection of thousands of bat samples from southern China to bring them back to Wuhan for study. The risks of such collection programs may outweigh the benefits.

A wiser, more practical choice might focus on detecting human spillover. That is biomedical surveillance. The pandemic spotlights the need for better surveillance and situational awareness about emerging infectious diseases, especially at the "One Health" interface where spillover events regularly occur.

Governments that care about health security have to develop a reasonable sense of what kind of work is going on, around the world, in all of these domains. The people who have this knowledge tend to work for a living on natural or synthetic biology, pharmaceuticals, healthcare, and veterinary biology. To know what is going on, governments need to build or tap into these networks of knowledge, across many countries.

Few intelligence analysts, and even fewer case officers in the U.S. government, have the scientific background to make much sense of what scientists, physicians, veterinarians, or pharmacists might be telling them. Therefore the U.S. government must decide where and how it wants to attract the experts on biological security who can provide the backbone for networks of situation awareness, the people who can translate situation awareness into actionable intelligence.

This point, by the way, is a basic reason for treating the Covid war as a global war, aside from the arguments of common humanity and common contagion. Governments that work globally, and earn global respect, will forge global connections and build a base of shared global knowledge.

Governments and labs in many countries have become naturally suspicious of scientists who want their interesting biological data. Genetic data or biological samples can earn recognition for foreign scientists or large profits for foreign pharmaceutical companies. Foreign authorities are looking for reciprocal relationships that can help them too.

The importance of situation awareness is one reason why it will turn out to be short-sighted if the United States is seen to have managed its Covid war in a way that ignored the rest of the world. Valued help earns respect and a seat at the lab bench.

The U.S. Centers for Disease Control and Prevention used to have quite a lot of global respect, global presence, and global networking. The CDC helped build programs to watch influenza and eradicate polio. CDC is still a very capable and respected institution. But CDC's overseas prestige and presence have ebbed. Now, organizations like France's Institut Pasteur or Germany's Robert Koch Institute or some experts at the World Health Organization may also be as well, or better, informed.

In the byzantine world of the immense U.S. Department of Defense, looking out for emerging infectious diseases that might endanger the "warfighter," there is a National Center for Medical Intelligence and overseas outposts of medical researchers. In the early 20th century, U.S. Army doctors, like Major Walter Reed, played a crucial role in suppressing tropical diseases like yellow fever to enable the building of the Panama Canal.

In today's military, the overseas outposts of military disease experts are usually associated with the U.S. Navy. Though they are a tiny part of the Pentagon's workforce, these operations are disproportionately important in the world of international disease surveillance. But they did not have the size or capability to be much help at the front end of the Covid war. The army has retained a role too, but the historically respected U.S. Army Medical Research Institute of Infectious Diseases was not authorized to apply its "biodefense" funding to the Covid war and it was sidelined early in the pandemic.

Much more valuable in the crisis was simply the large informal network of scientists and doctors working in hospitals and labs around the world, including networks connected through more influential nonprofit foundations. These relationships, often in academic medical and veterinary cooperation, have been mutually beneficial for years. For instance, since the level of expertise in some Chinese medical and research facilities is so high, their cooperation was invaluable in dealing with several past disease outbreaks. These relationships are fragile and vulnerable to Chinese Communist Party crackdowns. This sort of "scientist" or "doctor" diplomacy provided more valuable intelligence than anything else prior to and at the outset of the COVID-19 invasion.

The information from these informal networks has certainly been as good or better than the quality of intelligence or assessment available inside the U.S. government. It moves much faster than the process of writing and publishing scientific studies.

The world first received the genome for COVID-19 because of the quality of scientific cooperation between a Chinese scientist, Zhang Yongzhen, and an Australian scientist, Edward Holmes. Chinese and American doctors shared valuable clinical information during the crisis too. The politics of the Covid war have now constrained or shut down much exchange of knowledge in informal networks, especially as they connect to places like China or Russia.

China's failure to cooperate slowed warning about COVID-19 by at least several weeks. Chinese authorities failed to communicate the scale of the emerging pandemic, the risk to healthcare providers, and any early evidence of person-to-person transmission. Nor have they shared their own internal assessments of what really happened in Wuhan.

Some former U.S. health officials believe that some of their Chinese counterparts were also being kept in the dark or constrained by higher-level authorities. As late as mid-January 2020, Wuhan city briefings were still denying that there was "clear" evidence of any human-to-human transmissions. Among the first formal public releases from China of useful details about the disease, a January 20, 2020, field epidemiology report from a Chinese CDC team and a *Lancet* article posted four days later by national-level Chinese scientists, confirmed human-to-human transmission, community spread, some high degree of contagion, and a tentative but alarming initial *case* fatality rate of about 3 percent.[19] That is, 3 percent of patients with diagnosed cases died.

Though the Chinese did eventually share genetic sequences that kick-started early work on vaccines, they were not sharing actual viral specimens. This was a long-held tradition among virologists, stymied in this case. Such samples are vital to developing diagnostic tests and putting those tests through trials of effectiveness. So, other nations had to wait until some of their own citizens got sick.[20]

In 2005, after the first SARS, the countries of the world agreed on a revised set of International Health Regulations. These regulations required states to do more to detect and respond to outbreaks and warn the WHO about emerging health threats that might spread internationally. In the Covid war, this system failed. It failed because countries, including China, ignored these regulations and continued to ignore them throughout the pandemic response.

Those who want to improve this system of global biological intelligence will have to acknowledge that they cannot count on formal cross-national information sharing. The 2005 International Health Regulations system failed a crucial test. As a result, the World Health Organization, charged with overseeing that system on a basis of voluntary participation, also failed a crucial test.

More open societies will have to strengthen other global networks of people working on biological security. Most of those people will be motivated by common, cross-national interests, not just American interests, to understand what is going on and what is alarming. They will not be people just standing around and watching. They are more likely to be the people doing the work, the constructive, satisfying work investigating unusual outbreaks in humans or animals.

If governments do a better job of improving biomedical surveillance of human spillover events, growing the networks to do that, they still need to look harder at how that information will be consumed and shared. Covid demonstrated that even days of delay in action can have a huge effect on the trajectory of an emerging pandemic. We show how that story unfolded later in our report, in chapter 4, "Containment Fails; Mobilization Lags."

GOVERNING THE MOST RISKY RESEARCH

This war should prompt a massive, global effort to better regulate the most hazardous biological research. We think this is now essential. We understand that such regulation must strike a balance with progress in health research. We understand that not everyone will play by the rules. But paralysis is not the answer.

The bio revolution, including synthetic biology, will be one of the hallmarks of this era in world history. That was the role chemical engineering played in the late nineteenth and early twentieth century. It was the role physics and electrical engineering played in the second half of the last century and the early part of this one. In this era, potentially dangerous biological research is proliferating around the world, much of it in Asia.[21]

Though it can be immensely valuable, biological research can also threaten the health security of the world. The digital revolution has reduced the barriers of entry to high-end biological research. There is a huge amount of work going on. Quite a lot of that work is in Asia, not just in more traditional locations in North America, Europe, or Russia. The work goes on in many sectors, including biological, pharmaceutical, food, veterinary, and cosmetics research. The majority of the research is performed to develop commercial products. Therefore, a lot of the research is secretive and proprietary.

Some governments also maintain biological defense programs. Several governments worked on developing biological weapons before offensive work was banned by the 1972 Biological Weapons Convention. The Soviet government continued this work on a large scale, illegally, until a defector disclosed their programs to British and U.S. intelligence agencies in 1989. That discovery led to secret confrontations and, during the 1990s, a cooperative security program with the Russian government that shut the program down.[22]

The Russian government closed down or at least greatly reduced this program in the early 1990s, with much outside help. Outsiders never gained access to three of the critical defense ministry labs, and our group, at least, worries that the current Russian government may maintain a secret, illegal bioweapons program alongside its secret and illegal chemical weapons program. So far, the world's track record for regulating biological research is not encouraging.[23]

Any student of organizational culture and organizational safety has probably encountered a book by Charles Perrow, published in 1984, entitled *Normal Accidents: Living with High-Risk Technologies*. Perrow, a sociologist, observed that purely mechanical solutions to managing such technologies had become insufficient. The social systems to manage safe use of dangerous technologies were becoming so complex, and they interacted with each other in such byzantine ways, that failures were becoming more and more inevitable. Several major disaster investigations have underscored this insight.[24]

A major part of the Wuhan Institute of Virology and the China CDC's research missions was to prevent a future pandemic. The idea was that, by identifying viruses with the most spillover potential, and by identifying what kind of virus mixtures—"chimera" viruses—seemed dangerous, researchers could zero in on developing the specific drugs or vaccines that could neutralize them.

The Wuhan lab's program, and others like it, were being conducted by transnational groups of scholars from several countries. These research groups collected samples in various regions of the world. They studied them in multiple countries, including the United States. They were supported by several governments and foundations, including various agencies of the United States.

Nearly fifty years ago, in 1975, Paul Berg and Maxine Singer organized the Asilomar Conference on Recombinant DNA. They recognized that methods to alter and copy DNA sequences were about to become widely used in academic and industrial laboratories. They foresaw some of the risks. They emphasized treating biocontainment as part of experimental design, balancing risks. These principles are still followed in research, but the remarkable advances of the last half century call for a fresh reexamination of the deep issues at stake in synthetic biology.[25]

Long before the pandemic outbreak in Wuhan, the global scientific community had been debating the pros and cons of research programs that collect and experiment with potentially dangerous viruses, or experiment with them to explore their possible danger. Those debates have not been resolved. There are still no agreed upon international standards for what sorts of research would pass a risk-benefit test.

Any such standards would be technically complex and difficult to monitor across national borders. They must be written carefully so they do not inadvertently hinder necessary and beneficial research.

Nor are there adequate standards, across nations, to assure the biosafety of laboratories conducting necessary but dangerous research. It took about fifty years of large-scale industrial development to turn industrial safety into a science. Then industry complained that such work might hinder innovation or sacrifice competitive advantages. The science of industrial safety is now well developed. It is represented in the U.S. government by the National Institute for Occupational Safety and Health (NIOSH), which guides many laws, regulations, and insurance codes.

Although national, regional, and WHO initiatives exist, there is not yet any analogous scientific effort or institution for biosafety or standards for safe, secure biocontainment lab operations. This time, Americans and the world cannot afford to wait fifty years.

Early in 2020, China's armed forces conducted their own deep examination of what had gone wrong in Wuhan. As we mentioned, none of the results of this investigation have been made public. China also suffered a lab leak in 2019 at a veterinary vaccine company in Lanzhou, in northwest China, that resulted in thousands of people being infected with brucellosis, a bacterial illness with flu-like symptoms. Whatever the reason, in October 2020 the Chinese government chose to write and enact one of the most rigorous biosafety laws regulating laboratory work ever adopted by any country in the world. The U.S. should not be complacent; our country has had its own issues with biosafety.[26]

Beginning in 1946, countries have devoted enormous effort to control the dangers of atomic energy. They failed in some ways. But these efforts have succeeded more than most worried officials, in those early years, then thought possible. The biological challenge is probably more dangerous than the nuclear danger because bioweapons are harder to control, easier to make, and their effects can be more devastating. In some cases, creating biological weapons requires little skill, no technology, and no laboratory.

Biological hazards will definitely be more difficult to regulate globally. The relevant technology and materials are much more accessible. Businesses around the world are much more involved in the diffusion and use of biotech than was ever the case for atomic energy.

Analytically and institutionally, the regulatory challenge is intimidating. Yet experts must step up to show how such a regime must be devised and implemented. Practical planning must start with those governments that can bring the most knowledge, will, and ability to contribute.

Even if the world devises better regulations, that is not enough. Overseeing risky research relies on a leadership culture and individual researchers must accept this culture.

Labs with staff that have a strong safety culture, that don't view safety as a box-checking exercise, will be safer, more productive, and more rewarding places in which to work.

Writing regulations is actually the easy part. Implementing them effectively without slowing technical progress is more difficult, but it can be done by responsible leaders and researchers. Those leaders may not be biosafety experts, but they must genuinely accept responsibility for the security of their staff and the wider community. They must assemble, empower, and then support the technically qualified biosafety and operations team. They have to build an organizational culture of respect and trust in which there is a natural back and forth about safety worries.

These strategies—improved global situation awareness and governing the most risky research—can form real foundations of global, and American, intelligence about biological security. They can build stronger networks of knowledge about what is going on. But, if the United States government wants to make that case and build that capability, it must take these threats seriously and put in place competent technical leadership that can answer the "how" questions. It has to rebuild deep scientific expertise both at home and around the world.

3

THE DEFENDERS

THE UNITED STATES faced a twenty-first-century challenge with a system designed for nineteenth-century threats. Its national health security system was fundamentally designed circa 1890, in the administration of Grover Cleveland. Alarmed by outbreaks of cholera and typhoid in the fast-growing cities, state and local governments began establishing health departments, some even with their own laboratories, to apply science and sanitary hygiene to contain disease. One of the early leaders, a Massachusetts biologist, declared that "before 1880 we knew nothing; after 1890 we knew it all; it was a glorious ten years."[1]

By 1890, the advanced thinking about health security had two features. The state and local health departments were the first feature. They could call on the National Hygiene Laboratory, established in 1887.

The second feature was a federal service that mainly did medical inspections of incoming foreign ships and migrants. This started as the Marine Hospital Service, whose leaders developed the idea of a uniformed corps of public health physicians, a step signed into law by President Cleveland and later renamed the Public Health Service.

Local health departments had the job of spotting outbreaks and aggressively cleaning them up, often with fire
and bulldozer, as well as quarantining poor people and vaccinating them, sometimes forcibly. The public health innova-
tors of that era were committed to the new technology of
vaccination, especially against smallpox. They greatly, and
justifiably, feared the horrific death tolls suffered in the new
cities, like Chicago, from dirty water diseases like cholera or
typhoid, as well as the mosquito-borne diseases like yellow
fever. In the early twentieth century, having faced tropical
diseases in places like Cuba, the Philippines, and Panama,
the U.S. Army added more pathbreaking ideas and drive.

This health security design was characteristic of America's
other defenses, like its army. The United States had been
originally designed as a union of states. The states shouldered
most of the everyday burden to provide for the common
defense. Through much of its history, the peacetime army of
America's federal government was minuscule.

If some enemy appeared, state authorities would call up
local militias, organized by the states. Only in a really big
war would Congress authorize a suitable federal army. Then,
after that war, the federal army would deflate and disband.
What was left would be a small core of "regulars," to maintain some standards of leadership, training, and equipment.

The United States did not develop a larger peacetime
army, trained and equipped to federal standards, until after
it decided to join the First World War. The accompanying
great influenza pandemic of 1918–19 did not have a similar
effect on the health militias, however. The United States
never developed a state and federal reserve force, trained to
federal standards, to fight a biological invasion. The state and

local health departments remained America's nine-teenth-century-style health militias. The leaders were appointed in ways and on standards akin to the way state militia leaders were appointed in the 1890s.

The influenza crisis was, however, a great catalyst for scientific research. Following another influenza scare, in 1930 the National Hygiene Laboratory became the National Institute of Health (NIH). It later grew into a set of institutes. American society began relying on scientists to find the necessary miracle cures and vaccines. Then the system would help hand them out, as it would do after the development of influenza vaccines during the 1940s and polio vaccines during the 1950s.

Public health got its own research agency, originally called the Communicable Disease Center in the law passed in 1946. Located in Atlanta, because the South was the region with the most malaria, the institution evolved into a set of centers studying many topics from occupational health to infectious disease. Renamed the Centers for Disease Control and Prevention, it is more simply known as the CDC. It still had the job of gathering and studying up-to-date scientific information for the benefit of the state and local departments. Even as CDC evolved, the basic design was still in place. The executive agents—the policymaking decision makers who applied the knowledge in practice—were still the state and local health departments.

As the twentieth century wore on and the United States began developing a gigantic private healthcare industry, the old health militias became more and more anachronistic. Detached from the actual delivery of almost all healthcare, state and local health departments began devoting themselves instead to general prevention. Public health experts now refer to this period, through most of the twentieth century, as "Public Health 1.0."

By the 1980s, American public health experts believed the country was neglecting chronic disease and new threats, like the HIV/AIDS epidemic. They inaugurated a new era, which they called "Public Health 2.0," to professionalize the health departments, track chronic conditions, and study the social determinants of good health. They noted and decried the correlations of bad health with income or systematic disadvantage. They counseled schools and communities about their bad health habits, campaigning against smoking, venereal disease, and obesity. In the 2010s, advocates called for yet a further transition, to an era of "Public Health 3.0," in which communities would have a chief health strategist and work, across sectors, to build up "health, equity, and resilience in communities."[2]

THE OLD BONES

The net result is peculiar. Beyond the high ambitions, the bones of the American public health system are still the structure built for the challenges of the 1890s.

Nor are all the state and local health departments alike. In many states the state health department is dominant, centralizing all authority at the state level. But in many other states, the county or local departments are more powerful, decentralizing authority down to each local health jurisdiction. This "layered jurisdictional authority" forms a patchwork quilt of decentralized, detached, autonomous, and often contradictory operational plans and policies. No state and no local jurisdictions are the same. California's governance, for example, is quite fragmented—the counties are the main locus of authority, and their leadership varies enormously in background and skill.

The United States has twenty-eight hundred local public health departments, but these authorities are not organized into any coherent system. Half report to a centralized board of health; half do not. Some have carve-outs and carve-ins, where animal health is excluded but environmental health is included, and vice versa. No two are the same. Add to that antiquated information technology systems and it is no wonder that these departments cannot collect complete, reliable data on public health threats.

We are not saying that all the individual health departments are backward or anachronistic. Some are; some aren't. Some of their work is excellent. What we are saying is that the executive policymaking structure of health security still mainly resides in scores of state and local health departments analytically and institutionally.

We are also saying that these health departments remain fundamentally detached from the actual healthcare worlds of ordinary Americans. One reason why public health advice is more trusted in some countries is because they make wide use of community health workers in many different ways.[3]

Sometimes these community health workers are professionals; sometimes they are trained volunteers working with nonprofit or religious institutions. The main goals of such community health workforces are to try to reach citizens where they are, often with home visits, take a direct interest in their well-being, and help them connect to the wider healthcare system. These community workers become a personal bridge from public health to the healthcare system. People value the healthcare system because that is the system that helps them when they are sick.

The United States makes little use of community health workers who are directly connected to healthcare delivery. This is a structural weakness of the American system. By design, to avoid unwanted competition with for-profit services, such federal funds as exist for these programs are typically restricted to medically underserved areas eligible for a "federally qualified health center." These cover only about 9 percent of the population.[4]

As a result, these community health services and community health workers are seen as something for marginalized communities. That makes them low status. There is little recognition of their cost-effectiveness or political value.

The disconnect from the healthcare system handicaps the public health system in other ways. In the healthcare system, providers often have outstanding, twenty-first-century quality data about the operations in their own clinics and hospitals, as they have painfully improved the quality of their electronic health records. Providers with payment systems centered on patients, rather than fee-for-service, are nowadays commonly called "longitudinal care plans." The private operators of these longitudinal care plans have very good information about patient status and strong market incentives to reach out to them, including for preventive health.

But these data innovations, with their proprietary streams of electronic health records, are detached from the state, local, tribal, and territorial public health departments. Nor would private firms wish to share this data with such local

THE DEFENDERS * 59

agencies. The firms would not gain reciprocal insight that would help them care for patients and they would face proprietary and privacy risks. The public health entities try to get data in their own stream, with their own separate reporting requirements, with few resources to handle advanced data or deal with reluctant providers.

In 2019, just before the Covid war began, a group called the Council of State and Territorial Epidemiologists issued a report that few people noticed or read. This group represents the people in state and territorial health departments who are supposed to have intelligence, the situation awareness, about an emerging health danger.

Opening the report, the principal deputy director of the CDC, Anne Schuchat, asked whether their capabilities were more like "puttering along" in "our Model T Ford" or "speeding along in the latest electric car?" Her answer saw more kinship to the world of 1919 than the world of 2019. The key challenges the group then headlined, aside from the general lack of resources and expertise, were that, in 2019, "manual paper-based methods remain a prominent mode of data exchange"; updates happened in scores of individual efforts siloed from each other and not interoperable; and "a vast disconnect remains between health care and public health."[5]

In September 2022, the same systems were hampering America's response to an outbreak of mpox, formerly known as monkeypox. Frustrated by all the work-arounds in trying to make the Model T run, the new CDC director, Rochelle Walensky, lamented to a reporter that "if we have to reinvent the wheel every time we have an outbreak, we will always be months behind."[6]

Since public health departments do not provide health-care services, they find it challenging to persuade governments to give them enough money or qualified people. They usually do not employ an epidemiologist to investigate disease outbreaks except in cities and, even then, these are typically half-time positions. Even to provide basic public health services, outsiders judge that the departments are about eighty thousand staff short of what they need and have only about 60 percent of the required funds. Again, that is just to do the basics.[7]

For such departments, the panic of a health crisis can be a double-edged sword. They may get a rush of money for new hires. But they know that, when the crisis subsides, they will face a fiscal cliff with no likelihood that they can afford to keep these new people. Therefore, even in a crisis, the departments hesitate to invest in expanding their workforce.

Starved for funds from their home governments, many health departments look to federal grants to plug some of the gaps. The CDC is the conduit for a good portion of this federal money. Other HHS agencies and centers provide the rest. No one at HHS pulls all these streams together and clarifies overall strategic purpose to the recipients. The CDC funding formulas are byzantine, so complex that numbers of federal employees are required to figure out how to allocate the funds.

While public health departments in fifty states, four cities, and eight territories have received federal funding through the Public Health Emergency Preparedness (PHEP) program since 2002, this program does not make up for the fundamental neglect of core capabilities. It has not prepared these departments adequately for public health emergencies. Even this PHEP funding has dwindled. The program does not require recipients to maintain any level of preparedness, and, because no two health departments are alike, each uses the funds differently, often for programs that have little to do with preparedness. Tribal nations, some of which—like the Navajo Nation—had very high rates of Covid, were not eligible to apply for the PHEP.

The CDC influences a large part of the resources that flow to the front lines. Yet the CDC was never set up as an executive agency to orchestrate large-scale operations or deploy thousands of people in the field. It does not really manage pandemic preparedness and biodefense around America.

The executive agents were still supposed to be those state, local, territorial, and tribal health departments. The state, local, territorial, and tribal departments might have the nominal lead, but—except for mavericks like New York City—the departments have fallen into the habit of just looking for guidance from the CDC, an agency established for research and not equipped to provide executive leadership, nor equipped to manage the front lines of a nationwide battlefield.

THE NATIONAL PUBLIC HEALTH AGENCY— IMAGE AND REALITY

By the spring of 2020 and through the rest of that year, the six physicians most centrally involved in Washington's management of the Covid war were (in alphabetical order)

Deborah Birx, Anthony Fauci, Brett Giroir, Stephen Hahn, Robert Kadlec, and Robert Redfield. All had experience in the field of infectious disease and the challenge of combating outbreaks in the field. Both Birx and Redfield had also handled field clinical work in Africa; Birx in fact had come directly from Africa to serve, beginning in March 2020, as a coordinator of the White House Coronavirus Task Force.

In different ways and places, all have recounted their dismay with the CDC's inability to cross from its well-regarded research/investigational culture into the world of large operations. Birx was, at first, just bewildered by this, perhaps because she had been overseas so long. Redfield, on the other hand, had been the CDC's director for two years.

After he left office, trying to help congressional investigators understand his concerns, Redfield recounted how, in his first briefing as the CDC director in 2018, he had asked about opioid-related deaths. "'[W]hat was the data through?' And the briefer, with a straight face, told me, 'March 2015.' And I said, 'But it's April 2018.' And he said, 'Director, you don't understand the complexity of getting data from the states and assimilating it.'"[8]

Redfield replied: "When I came here [to] the premier public health agency of the world . . . I thought I was coming down here to use data to make an impact on public health. And you're telling me what I really am is, I'm a medical historian."

To Redfield, "The culture of the agency is not a response agency. It's a 'we collect data, and tell you what happened.' . . . And most of the people at CDC, which I respect, but they've [been] lull[ed] into feeling like they're in academic

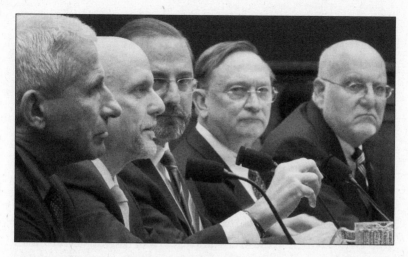

Department of Health and Human Services officials testify to Congress about the coronavirus on February 26, 2020. *From left:* NIAID Director Anthony Fauci, FDA Commissioner Stephen Hahn, HHS Secretary Alex Azar, ASPR Robert Kadlec, and CDC Director Robert Redfield. PHOTO CREDIT: CHIP SOMODEVILLA/ GETTY IMAGES

medical science, an Emory [University] II." And still, in 2022, Redfield believed that "we don't have an integrated system [for public health data] in this country."

When he was interviewed by the House subcommittee investigating the Covid crisis, Giroir had been the assistant secretary of health in the Department of Health and Human Services for about three years, 2018–21. A lifelong student of infectious disease, he had gone from treating children to academia, then was one of the first physicians to hold a managerial role at the Defense Advanced Research Projects Agency (DARPA), then he went back to academia, and on to the private sector. In his last job he had overseen the Public Health Service and worked closely with the CDC.

"I'm going to start at a macro level," Giroir explained. "I think there's two fundamental problems . . . and they're linked."[9]

"The CDC," he went on, "has become like an independent academic institution in their ivory tower. They have almost no urgency and almost zero operational capability. And that was shown in the pandemic." He was bewildered to see CDC trying "to improve maternal health . . . and have a thousand people working on that, which is really HRSA's role [the Health Resources and Services Administration of HHS]," at which HRSA was the best, "bar none." The CDC had to focus on its core mission. It needed "to understand how to control infectious disease."

Giroir found the situation tragic because "CDC is a great organization. . . . The people at CDC are generally excellent. The culture of the institution needs to be completely, you know, refitted and redone."

Giroir then turned to his second critique, which he had learned from his budget work. Even if CDC tried to reform, so much of what it did was administer programs and processes mandated by Congress, with little discretion to make policy. "Everything is so compartmentalized that there's very little flexibility in the CDC budget, and there's really not a whole lot of flexible money at the CDC director's level."

The CDC was fractured into too many missions. For instance, he said, the CDC found itself funding the vital and neglected work on community health centers, while "the CDC needs to focus on global epidemics." Redfield made the same point. His organization had more than ten thousand people. But he had to manage "a jillion different independently funded projects by Congress that I had very little flexibility with."

An organization's culture is closely related to what its people are asked to do every day. Take, for instance, the issue of controlling infectious disease. The CDC does have an operational capability—to handle quarantines and investigate outbreaks with great skill. This capability has long been structured for small outbreaks, like an Ebola patient landing in the United States. The CDC could send scores of people to manage this. It could work with the State Department and the Department of Homeland Security to rearrange flights from a part of Africa. It could be sure that state public health labs could test for such an exotic disease, on a scale of dozens or perhaps hundreds of samples. But it was not structured or oriented for large-scale challenges, either at home or overseas.

The deep issue is that the CDC's culture reasonably reflects the role and missions Congress has granted to it. Congress has done this mainly through many programs, not any overarching legislative design. CDC lives and breathes inside the old bones of the original nineteenth-century design. Most of the executive and operational authorities, most of the trained manpower and equipment, are not in CDC. They are in the thousands of state, local, territorial, and tribal militias.

This reality clashes not only with CDC's public image, but even with its image of itself. As director Redfield has put it, the CDC was "the premier public health agency." But, in many operational ways, not really.[10]

The abilities are there. The Covid war generated a striking illustration of what is possible. In the first chapter, where we spotlighted the unheralded executive competence, we mentioned the annual awards given out by Max Stier and the nonprofit Partnership for Public Service. In 2022, one of those awardees was the CDC's Anita Patel.

During Operation Warp Speed, which we will say more about later, Patel—a pharmacist—was a key member of the team that worked out the blueprints for how hundreds of millions of Covid vaccines could be distributed in an unprecedented partnership with private pharmacy chains like CVS and Walgreens. A private consultant observed that "[t]he federal-pharmacy partnership expanded the public health infrastructure of the U.S. by threefold in about two days." Almost all the U.S. population lives within a few miles of a pharmacy. A division director in another part of HHS noted: "If you got your vaccine in a pharmacy, it's because of the work Anita Patel did."[11]

THE NATIONAL HEALTH SECURITY ENTERPRISE—IMAGE VERSUS REALITY

When the Covid war began, Anne Schuchat was still the number two person at the CDC. She was the most senior career official in the agency, highly respected, and with thirty-two years of service. She was realistic about what CDC could and could not do. From her point of view, CDC, and all the public health departments, were just one section of the orchestra.

Early in the pandemic, in February 2020, she recalled to congressional investigators that CDC already had its own task forces trying to keep up with the data about the outbreak. They were talking to foreign counterparts. They were working with the airlines and others in the federal government to channel travel from China, screen incoming travelers, organize small quarantine efforts, and develop a Covid test (which CDC did very quickly, but then adopted a flawed design for producing it).

Schuchat was looking to others to put all this in the context of a larger policy design for coping with a potential pandemic. She was looking ahead to the large policy issues already apparent, including "what are we going to tell schools, universities, and businesses?"[12]

She continued: "And all these issues having reached the next trigger, we were trying to queue up the planning for community mitigation . . . our efforts to delay the spread. We were trying to queue up the healthcare preparedness in terms of PPE [personal protective equipment] and reusables. And what was the strategy to get enough where we knew we didn't have enough supply." These issues were outside of CDC.

"And then, of course . . . we were not ready for a very large-scale quarantine effort either at the federal level or at the state level. We didn't have the systems. We didn't have the people. We didn't have the technology [to track cases and get needed information from the airlines], or the agreement on [using] the technology to do that in a swift and efficient way."

From her point of view, those and other big policy choices "couldn't get onto the agenda at the HHS or NSC meetings because most of the conversations were: 'How are we going to deal with [the latest] batch of cruise ship people?' . . . We didn't have the right policy governance to get the key issues escalated and decisions made."

Her bottom line was that "I think during this relatively chaotic period there wasn't strategic-level governance." She never saw an adequate institution to do the policy designs.

Imagine the national health security enterprise as an orchestra. An orchestra has four usual sections—strings, woodwinds, brass, and percussion. But they only play well if enabled by common sheet music and a conductor.

What Schuchat calls "strategic-level governance" provides the conductor and the sheet music that designate each section's role and what notes to play. In health security, the sections that have to play in harmony include, at the very least,

- the public health community (CDC and the thousands of health departments);

- the healthcare system (public and private); and

- the biopharma system (public and private) for developing and deploying tests, drugs, and vaccines.

And, while they are playing their instruments, all of these sections have to monitor their performance: the public health community tracking outbreaks with help from the healthcare system; the healthcare system forming networks to track their capacity and the success of clinical treatments; and the biopharma system analyzing the biology of possible diagnostics, therapies, and vaccines.

Still, at the center of the enterprise, someone needs to write the common sheet music and conduct the orchestra. At the beginning of 2020, the U.S. government did not have either a composer or a conductor.

A national health security enterprise would have executive leadership to map out the overall strategy, the "how," as it sized up the danger and the availability of countermeasures. Such leadership would communicate clear, credible messages about the situation. Such leadership would also balance public health requirements with practical and social issues, linked with how leaders sized up their instruments for treatment, screening, drugs, or vaccines.

During the Covid war that leadership started with the office of the secretary of Health and Human Services (HHS). That was an appropriate place to look for it. The president of the United States and White House staff were obviously important. But daily operational leadership had to come from a line organization, connected to Congress, and with people in the field.

The HHS secretary has traditionally been viewed as the head of a domestic welfare department, running Medicare and Medicaid, and loosely supervising autonomous bastions for research (NIH), drug safety (FDA), and the CDC. For more than ten years, as the implementation of the Affordable Care Act has evolved, the great bastion of supervision over the healthcare system has, even more than before, become CMS, the Centers for Medicare and Medicaid Services. The head of CMS is regarded by some insiders as more powerful than the secretary of HHS. The secretariat of HHS did not have the experience, or the operational culture, to prepare it to manage a national health security emergency.

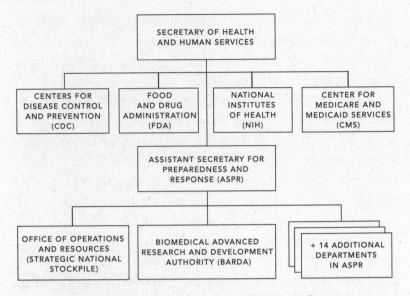

An abbreviated Department of Health and Human Services organizational chart reflecting key players in the federal response to the COVID-19 pandemic. In early 2020, CDC, FDA, NIH, and CMS were four of the eleven operating divisions. At the time, ASPR, which is responsible for BARDA and the Strategic National Stockpile, was a staff division in the office of the HHS secretary. ASPR was elevated to an operating division in July 2022 and renamed the Administration for Strategic Preparedness and Response.

Our group proposes a different conception for the proactive, strategic leadership of a national health security enterprise. The current system may seem like a balance of federal, state, and local authorities. In practice, it is a recipe for dysfunction.

- It is unbalanced because the public health enterprise is not truly "federal" or "national." It concentrates almost all operational responsibility at the state, local, territorial, and tribal levels. The federal authorities offer detached guidelines and pass along money in an elaborate grants process, which almost guarantees that the first will be ineffectual and the second will be inefficient.

- Meanwhile, the current system is also unbalanced because the healthcare system, and its information and emergency readiness, are detached from the public health enterprise.

- Then the current system is unbalanced still more because the mustering of big medical counter-measures—tests, drugs, and vaccines—is not only detached from the public health enterprise and the CDC, but is weak inside HHS itself, with little peacetime capacity to proactively build the public-private partnerships that will be needed in an emergency.

We value America's layered federal system, leaning on the insights and judgment of those who are closest to what is going on. Federalism is an asset. There is no great need for powerful new federal legal authorities. As we will point out, the latent authorities of HHS are already strong, especially in CMS.

We imagine a system of national health security in which information is networked and operations are distributed, but there is national executive leadership, aided by a much stronger core of trained, deployable public health regulars. Only national executive leadership can orchestrate real strategies to contain an outbreak and deploy the toolkits of counter-measures to help communities defend themselves.

Within the United States, both situation awareness and fielding countermeasures will roll down to state and local operations. Those will often need their own public-private partnerships. The countermeasures and the supply chains to produce them not only need national management, but also international coalition strategy to deal with multinational conglomerates and their suppliers or distribution networks.

In our vision, the "vast disconnect" between public health and healthcare systems would close. On the front lines, the successful ad hoc combinations of agencies and local stake-holders during the Covid war, often put together by gover-nors and mayors, would turn into peacetime institutions with habits of real-time data sharing, health security updates, and coordinated readiness to handle surges and emergencies, reg-ularly practiced. National leadership has a role to play not just in offering general medical advice of how to stay safe, but in providing practical suggestions of how to do it, and commu-nicate about it, taking all the relevant issues into account.

In this vision, a changed CDC still has a vital role that plays to its core strength of tracking and analyzing, in real time, what is going on—the hub of a national network of state, local, and tribal health departments in the field, better linked to local healthcare providers. For this data sharing to work, CMS may need to develop an alternative to relying on state health departments as its regulatory enforcers. Health-care companies will be reluctant to link real-time data flows to their regulators.

The executive policymaking mission cannot be in the CDC. It must be closer to centers of federal leadership to orchestrate the skills, concerns, and policy instruments, including logistics and procurement, that go beyond the usual training of medical doctors and epidemiologists.

Our alternative vision grows out of what we saw and experienced during the Covid war. It also grows, though, out of what we remember about the years before the war began.

THE AFTERMATH OF 9/11

The first real challenge to the anachronistic structure of the American health security system came after September 11, 2001. This trauma became the public health system's "First World War" wake-up call. In October 2001, a terrorist mailed anthrax spores to victims (eventually attributed to a rogue American scientist who took his own life). That scare was followed by many others. There were alarms about terrorist interest in bioweapons, coming on top of the 1990s-era disclosures about the scope of the Soviet Union's illegal bioweapons program.

At that moment, one of us, John Barry, happened to publish his history of the great influenza pandemic. It was a powerful reminder about the scale of natural dangers, like another, and even deadlier, global flu outbreak.

President George W. Bush read Barry's book. The resulting flow of funds caused people to tell us that Barry had written the "seven-billion-dollar book." This preparedness agenda was codified in the National Strategy for Pandemic Influenza in November 2005 and its corresponding Implementation Plan in May 2006, which detailed a whole-of-government response to a future influenza pandemic.[13]

Many American veterans of pandemic preparedness are a bit nostalgic about the period between 2005 and 2010. They look back on it as a relative high-water mark. Some of this promise was structural. There was a new assistant secretary for Preparedness and Response (the ASPR, always pronounced "asper") in the Department of Health and Human Services (HHS). The ASPR oversaw the new Biomedical Advanced Research and Development Authority (BARDA) to develop life-saving drugs or vaccines.

The ASPR also oversaw the Strategic National Stockpile of needed supplies, a program originally managed by the CDC. The stockpile emphasized countermeasures to established dangers like anthrax, smallpox, and especially bird flu. There was less emphasis on other kinds of medical supplies.

These structures combined with the capabilities of the new Department of Homeland Security (DHS) and a dedicated White House office concerned with pandemic readiness. More important was a surge of capable new people who, armed with the new money, took the danger very seriously and together prepared hard for it. They shared a common sense of roles, mission, and urgency.

In 2006, HHS established the Public Health Emergency Medical Countermeasures Enterprise. (PHEMCE, usually pronounced "fem-see"). It was designed to coordinate preparedness across the U.S. government.

A 2009 alarm about a possible H1N1 flu epidemic brought the parties together and demonstrated this readiness. It also revealed continuing weaknesses. The government had been lucky in that case, one participant thankfully recalled. "We didn't dodge a bullet; nature shot us with a BB gun."

PANIC, THEN NEGLECT

Even that limited readiness faded in the following ten years. The public pronouncements sounded fine. In his 2010 State of the Union address, President Obama called for "a new initiative that will give [the United States] the capacity to respond faster and more effectively to bioterrorism or an infectious disease—a plan that will counter threats at home and strengthen public health abroad." In 2012, the PHEMCE "strategy" promised a "nimble, flexible capacity to produce medical countermeasures rapidly in the face of any public health attack or threat, known or unknown."[14]

The programs sounded fine. The Obama administration, for example, established and spent several hundred million dollars on Centers for Innovation in Advanced Development and Manufacturing (CIADMs), which would produce the drugs or vaccines that the private sector would not, and spent more money on "fill-finish" facilities to package the doses. But these centers needed peacetime work to keep the lights on. Unless they had well-trained people doing quality work in peacetime, the operators could not quickly ramp them up, find all the people, meet quality standards, and produce for wartime.

The Covid war would later prove that point. Some of these facilities did not help at all and even backfired (assigned to produce many doses, then failed, with all the work lost). Some of the investments helped, but they did not add much to the U.S. and European capacity to produce drugs or vaccines during the crisis.

By 2019, after ten years of strategy and program pronouncements, it was more and more clear that the operational structures for a bio emergency would not be ready for one. The Trump administration's ASPR was Robert Kadlec. Kadlec had been a career physician in the U.S. Air Force, retiring as a colonel after work as a flight surgeon. He then held several jobs dealing with biodefense in the Pentagon, in the George W. Bush White House, and in the Senate.

As the ASPR, Kadlec was a staff adviser to the HHS secretary, Alex Azar. His office was not regarded as an operational division. It "did policy," drafting strategies, for example. The ASPR office thus had little executive authority of its own, and certainly none over the big players even housed in its own HHS department, like the National Institutes of Health or the Food and Drug Administration. As for day-to-day leadership of America's public health community, the CDC thought that was its job.

The real emergency management muscle, not just in Washington but across the country, was in another department. It was in the Department of Homeland Security, in its Federal Emergency Management Agency (FEMA). While equipped to deal with domestic disasters like hurricanes and earthquakes, which are usually confined to a particular area and of relatively short duration, FEMA was not structured to handle a rolling, nationwide crisis spanning years. Nor did it have the expertise to combat outbreaks of infectious disease.

What FEMA did have was money. Its Disaster Relief Fund started the 2020 fiscal year with more than $29 billion in available reserves (budgeters call these "unobligated balances"). These funds can be tapped after the president declares an emergency or major disaster under the Stafford Act. President Trump did that on March 13, 2020.[15]

That disaster money could then flow to all sorts of emergency assistance purposes, staffed from whatever U.S. agency was needed. By the end of March, Congress began opening floodgates of money.

But by the end of March, the mobilization was already running about two months behind, and it still took time to organize and deploy meaningful help. We will comment later on the substance of the FEMA work, because FEMA also brought some notable operational strengths—and weaknesses—to the crisis. Here we only echo a comment one of us made, a physician who handled emergency cases during the pandemic. His firsthand observation was that "by the time FEMA arrived, the ballgame was over."

If FEMA was not enough, there was the military—in yet another department. That was a last resort in a national emergency. During the Covid war, that point arrived in the spring of 2020.

As the post-9/11 panic faded, the readiness money ebbed and the stockpiles aged. Worries about biodefense against rogue states, like North Korea, tended to push aside worries about a natural pandemic.

In the Trump administration, after a long bureaucratic struggle, HHS moved responsibility for the Strategic National Stockpile away from CDC and gave it to the ASPR, to Kadlec. As Scott Gottlieb, who at the time was the head of the FDA, recounts in his book: "Once the stockpile was moved under the ASPR, its primary mission would predictably evolve, with more emphasis put on the risks posed by biological weapons and less on pandemics."[16]

The Trump National Security Council staff (during John Bolton's tenure as national security advisor) closed its pandemic preparedness office. The tasks were moved around. The symbolism of the separate office was less important than having high-powered talented people working on the health security problem. The White House lost a couple of capable executives with deep health security experience and it was hard to replace them.

Structures still existed on paper. In addition to the Public Health Service's Commissioned Corps, the United States had a National Disaster Medical System (NDMS), mainly in name only—more readiness for hurricanes. The ASPR supposedly guided the Medical Reserve Corps to organize local volunteers to help with local events. But the ASPR did not control the funds. Those were non-federal. The volunteers never attained the numbers nor received the training to be relied on as a medical reserve corps when crisis arrived.

Congress passed the Pandemic and All Hazards Preparedness Act in 2006. It passed the Reauthorization Act of the same name in 2013. It passed the Pandemic and All Hazards Preparedness and Advanced Innovations Act in 2019. More "programs," hollow in relation to what was coming.

There was the Public Health Emergency Fund, created in 1983 to have flexible money ready for an emergency. In 2016, for example, responding to the Zika virus scare, Representative Rosa DeLauro (D-CT) had urged that $5 billion be placed in this fund, so the money would be ready right away if something happened. She and others kept pressing this cause. But in 2019, when the Covid invasion hit, the fund had less than $60,000.[17]

There was the Infectious Disease Rapid Response Reserve Fund. Going into 2020, HHS might tap about $105 million. That amount, a few months later, would turn out to be a tiny fraction of what the "infectious disease rapid response" rapidly needed to spend.[18]

There was a new Executive Order, signed by President Trump, about how to get ready for a big influenza outbreak. The language of the order was good. But there was no money behind it—none. Just words.[19]

Back in November 2016, President Obama's science advisers had given him a dire warning. Despite his pronouncements during the last eight years, they said "immediate action" was needed to strengthen biodefenses. They remembered some recent scares, including an outbreak of Ebola virus in Africa.[20]

The White House official who eventually led that Ebola response was Ron Klain. He served as President Joe Biden's chief of staff until early 2023. He wrote, in 2016, that "the next President must act from Day One" to prepare for a far more threatening test of global health systems that was on the horizon. "If she or he waits until grim-faced aides file into the Oval Office to explain that a pandemic is unfolding, it will be far too late to save countless people around the world, protect our interests abroad, and preserve lives here at home."[21]

Experts both outside and inside of the government knew that the system, from top to bottom, was unready for a pandemic. They wrote reports calling attention to some of the deficits. In September 2019, just before the Covid outbreak, the White House Council of Economic Advisers issued its own little-noticed report. It estimated that a pandemic (influenza, for example) would cause economic damage that could range from nearly half a trillion to nearly four trillion dollars. It thought, if the pandemic was really bad, it could kill more than half a million people.[22]

That 2019 report may have seemed alarmist. It actually greatly *under*estimated the impact of what was about to hit.

Even the ASPR himself, Kadlec, openly described how the federal system had deteriorated. Speaking in October 2018 to a group of students at the University of Texas, Kadlec warned them: "If we don't build this" readiness hedge against a pandemic, "we're gonna be SOL [shit out of luck] should we ever be confronted with it."[23]

Kadlec did not have to wait long to be proven right. On the morning of January 28, 2020, the picture Ron Klain had painted in his warning essay of 2016 came to life: the "grim-faced aides" did indeed "file into the Oval Office to explain that a pandemic was unfolding." It did indeed turn out to be "far too late to save countless people around the world, protect our interests abroad, and preserve lives here at home."

4

CONTAINMENT FAILS; MOBILIZATION LAGS

═══

JOSHUA SHARFSTEIN IS a professor of public health at Johns Hopkins University who first worked as a pediatrician and eventually became the health commissioner of Baltimore before serving as principal deputy at the FDA. Sharfstein penned a book for his students called *The Public Health Crisis Survival Guide*. In that book, after describing a crisis he faced in Baltimore, he writes that the crisis taught him "a key lesson: The first order of business in crisis management is figuring out that there is a crisis."[1]

Part of the challenge of analyzing the U.S. response to the Covid war is determining when those in key positions of authority figured out that there was, in fact, a crisis. When did they realize that a war was upon them?

There are two main kinds of military history books. One kind recounts the human experience of battles and war zones. These books vividly recall explosions, bullets cracking overhead, traumatic scenes, people ducking and yelling as they fight or are struck down. They depict a range of human behavior, from heroic to squalid. We are fortunate that there are already at least half a dozen such books, good ones, on the sound and fury of the Trump administration's Covid war, especially the Trump White House, without even counting the memoirs and testimonies.[2]

The other kind of military histories analyzes why battles, campaigns, or wars turned out the way they did, perhaps to draw out lessons. That is our approach.

Stepping back, analyzing the outset of this war, the month of January 2020 was a month of warnings and early reactions. February was a month in which some nations mobilized and the United States did not. American leaders quarreled about what was going on, what to say about it, or how to try to keep it away. The virus was spreading rapidly in parts of the United States during March and a bewildering set of emergency responses began.

FIRST WARNINGS

On New Year's Eve, 2019, China CDC director George Gao spoke with the leader of one of the most important nonprofit foundations working on global health, Britain's Wellcome Trust. He told this leader, Jeremy Farrar, about some cases of a new pneumonia in Wuhan. Gao said it was not SARS (the syndrome that had crossed over from animals in 2002–04). CDC director Robert Redfield also spoke with Gao on New Year's Eve and on through the following week.[3]

In both those initial calls, Gao said he did not see evidence of human-to-human transmission in an initial set of twenty-seven cases, all of which had, he thought, been related to a "wet market," a wildlife market in Wuhan. In a follow-up with Redfield, two or three days later, Gao described family clusters of cases, which implied human-to-human transmission.

Redfield was also puzzled about the "case definition"—as some sort of "unspecified pneumonia" related to the wet market. He recalled for Gao mistakes in case definition Americans had made about HIV/AIDS. They had focused only on certain kinds of people, because those people had surfaced as the initial cases. He encouraged Gao to check for such pneumonia cases outside the wet market.

A couple of days later, Gao spoke again to Redfield. "He said," Redfield later told congressional investigators, "he did look outside, and there's hundreds of cases. And they had nothing to do with the wet market."

Gao was plainly now quite worried. Redfield respected Gao's ability and integrity. Gao was an expert on coronaviruses. Redfield later concluded that Gao was sharing what he knew and, at that point, Gao was not much better informed about what was happening in Wuhan than Redfield was.[4]

Redfield was also in frequent contact with the head of the World Health Organization, Tedros Adhanom Ghebreyesus, a physician and former Ethiopian minister of health and of foreign affairs. Redfield knew Tedros from common field work in Africa. Both Redfield and Tedros offered to send CDC and WHO teams to China immediately, to help investigate the outbreak. This was not unusual. What was unusual was that the Chinese government steadily refused all such offers in those early weeks.

By early January 2020, many outsiders were picking up signs of alarm among Chinese doctors and municipal officials in Wuhan. The Chinese government was starting to control communications about the crisis, while organizing exceptional efforts to contain an apparent outbreak.

By the middle of January, outside experts knew they were dealing with a novel coronavirus. At first some would say it had "SARS-like" qualities, a potentially misleading label, since the earlier SARS had not spread in the same way and had few asymptomatic cases.

One set of alarmed people consisted of informal networks of scientists and doctors, including many members of our group. One of these circles, some of whom had worked together in the Bush 43 administration, jokingly called themselves the "Wolverines," echoing the label of an underground resistance group in the Reagan-era movie *Red Dawn*. Farrar was plugged into these networks. On the inside of the government, so was the ASPR, Kadlec.[5]

HHS leaders were following the outbreak in China. They kept working, unsuccessfully, to get a CDC team in, both to help and to share understanding of what was happening.

One of Kadlec's deputies was Rick Bright, a longtime civil servant who headed BARDA, the office in the ASPR that interfaced with private industry to develop life-saving drugs or vaccines. In mid-January, Bright returned from the annual J.P. Morgan Healthcare Conference in San Francisco, where it had seemed like everyone was talking about the virus. Back in his office, with his team Bright drew up a

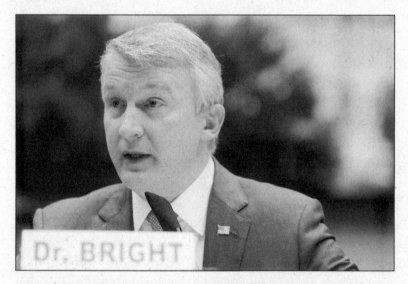

Rick Bright, former Biomedical Advanced Research and
Development Authority director, testifies to Congress on May 14,
2020. Bright had filed a federal whistleblower complaint the
previous week, after being forced out as BARDA's director.
PHOTO CREDIT: GREG NASH-POOL/GETTY IMAGES

notional "horse race" on his whiteboard of a portfolio of several companies for possible crash simultaneous investment in
vaccines and drugs.

In the third week of January, Bright started calling company leaders at Johnson & Johnson, Roche, Pfizer, Genen-
tech, Regeneron, and the small new company they had helped
to support, called Moderna, discussing what they would need
in a crisis mobilization. He was also talking to possible suppliers of vials, like Corning, or a manufacturer of N95 masks,
Prestige Ameritech. The CEO of Prestige Ameritech had long

been worried about crisis supplies and could see surging demand in Asia. He pleaded with officials to make a large, urgent effort to secure U.S. supply lines and open new ones. On January 20, an infectious disease expert (and member of our group), Michael Osterholm, sounded the pandemic alarm to a top executive at a big manufacturer of N95s based in his home state, Minnesota. The executive was convinced. To its credit, 3M had prepared to make more masks in the United States if there was a crisis.[6]

The well-connected outsider, Farrar at the Wellcome Trust, realized that Chinese authorities were not disclosing all they knew about the crisis to the World Health Organization. On January 18, Farrar received an alarm from a Dutch scientist who was reviewing a Chinese paper on the virus that would be published in the *Lancet* on January 24. That paper made it clear that the virus had human-to-human transmission and that some infected people were asymptomatic.[7]

The first cases of COVID-19 were only just beginning to show up in foreign countries. On January 20, the first case was confirmed in the United States, in Seattle. In fact, as would become clear much later, many cases had arrived in the United States, and not just in Seattle. But those early American cases were asymptomatic or they went unrecognized as an "influenza-like illness."

On January 22, Farrar received projections from one of the Wolverines (and a member of our group), Carter Mecher, that "this is taking off faster than SARS." The next day Mecher warned that we were "not going to be able to outrun it." Mecher wrote: "Two weeks from now, are there things that we wished we could have done to reshape the challenge we will likely face?"

On January 25, Farrar began telling colleagues: "This cannot be contained in China and will become a global pandemic over the next few days/weeks of uncertain severity. Since influenza 1918 things have never turned out quite as bad as they appear early on . . . but this is the first time since SARS I have been worried."[8]

THINK 1918

In the last week of January 2020, the two lead figures in the White House most closely watching the spreading virus outbreak were the chief of the Domestic Policy Council, Joe Grogan, a veteran of the health policy and pharma world, and the deputy national security advisor, Matt Pottinger. For different reasons, talking to different people, both were growing more and more concerned about the crisis.

Even before the crisis, Grogan regarded the HHS secretary, Alex Azar, as a disaster. Azar regarded Grogan as a cancer. Pottinger shared the general White House lack of trust in Azar. On Monday, January 27, the White House acting chief of staff, Mick Mulvaney, asked Grogan and Pottinger to organize more work on the unfolding crisis.

Pottinger, like some of his White House colleagues, was already deeply suspicious about the Chinese government. Pottinger had covered the earlier SARS crisis, in China, as a young reporter for the *Wall Street Journal*, and his wife worked in public health.[9] Over the weekend Pottinger had reached out to Chinese experts. Early on Tuesday morning, January 28, while driving to work at the White House, Pottinger received what he described to us as "the most important phone call I had ever received." It was, he said, from an unimpeachable source, a highly qualified doctor treating patients and visiting hospitals in China. The doctor was recounting facts that were already weeks old.

The doctor told Pottinger that the virus was in uncontrolled community spread in China, in multiple provinces. Fifty percent of the cases were asymptomatic, the doctor said, and asymptomatic carriers were spreading the virus. Trying to take this in, Pottinger asked if this was as bad as SARS, the outbreak that Pottinger had covered as a young journalist, nearly twenty years earlier. "Forget SARS," the doctor replied. "Think 1918." It was the big one.

Pottinger immediately briefed his boss, the national security advisor, Robert O'Brien. O'Brien asked Pottinger to attend President Trump's the President's Daily Brief (PDB) that morning.

The Covid crisis was not the top item in that morning's PDB. When the briefer, Beth Sanner, got to that item, O'Brien said, "This will be the biggest national security threat you face in your presidency."

President Trump pursued this with the briefer. She said the intelligence community did not have enough information to draw firm conclusions, but it looked like it might not be as bad as the earlier SARS outbreak. O'Brien pushed back: "This is going to be the roughest thing you face." Pottinger then jumped in to agree, standing up to make his point.

Pottinger told the president what he had learned. Unlike SARS, this virus appeared to have rapid human-to-human spread, much of it asymptomatic, and it had already spread far and fast. It was probably already en route to the United

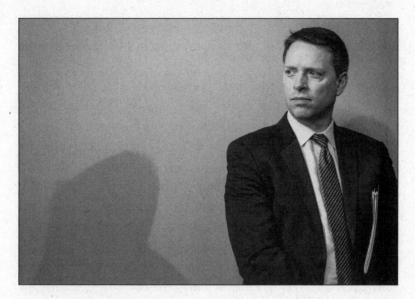

Matthew Pottinger, Assistant to the President and Deputy National Security Advisor, listening at the White House press briefing on the coronavirus on January 31, 2020. PHOTO CREDIT: JABIN BOTSFORD/THE WASHINGTON POST VIA GETTY IMAGES

States. Asked what to do, Pottinger started with a suggestion to cut off travel from China to the United States.

After the briefing, Pottinger told us that Mulvaney, who had been there, was "incandescent with anger." Mulvaney asked Pottinger if he thought he was the head of HHS or the CDC and berated him as out of line for proposing a travel shutdown.

That afternoon, Pottinger convened an NSC meeting and included, as a bureaucratic ally, Peter Navarro. Navarro, an economist known for his all-out emphasis on the China threat, had been in the Trump administration from day one. With a well-earned reputation as an abrasive bureaucratic bomb-thrower, Navarro had antagonized Mulvaney and most others on the White House team, but President Trump liked him.

After the NSC meeting, Pottinger relayed what he had learned from China to a small group, including Azar, Anthony Fauci, and Redfield. Fauci was skeptical of the account, believing that, from his experience, this was not how respiratory viruses operated. The message from Fauci and Redfield was to wait for more information before sounding a full alarm—the risk to the United States was still low.

That same day, January 28, the *Wall Street Journal* ran an op-ed piece entitled "Act Now to Prevent an American Epidemic." It was by Luciana Borio and Scott Gottlieb. Borio had been the acting chief scientist of the FDA during the Obama administration. She had then served until 2019 on the Trump administration's NSC staff, handling medical and biodefense policy. Gottlieb had headed the FDA in the Trump administration until the previous year. He was estranged from Azar, but had been regularly texting his concerns to Grogan.[10]

Borio and Gottlieb were already looking past travel bans. They were, quite rightly, pressing for broadly conceived strategies of emergency readiness: mass testing to detect spread and preparations for hospitals to get ready. Like Bright in BARDA, they too were already calling for a crash program to develop vaccines and drugs, to start lining up people for the coming clinical trials.

Also that day, back at HHS, both Kadlec, the ASPR, and Giroir, the assistant secretary of health, received an email from an American doctor, Michael Callahan (a member of our group), who had just been treating patients in Wuhan.

Callahan reported that the virus was spreading fast. The virus, which lingered in those infected and asymptomatic, and in minimally ill people, "will propagate virus into distant communities." Callahan could not yet tell how deadly the virus might be, except that he could see it was worse than seasonal flu.[11]

By the next day, Mulvaney had created the White House Coronavirus Task Force. Limiting Pottinger's role, Mulvaney put Azar in charge of the task force. He detailed Grogan to be part of it too. Pottinger and Navarro were so insistent about sounding the alarm that, after the first meeting, Mulvaney asked O'Brien to "get Pottinger under control" and he kicked Navarro off the task force. Navarro then, as was his habit, circulated a memo, dated January 29, to warn that America was defenseless against the danger of a "full-blown pandemic" that might inflict several trillion dollars in damages and kill more than half a million people.

That Navarro, an economist, was making this argument did not help make it more credible to those health experts who were still on the fence. They still thought the outbreak posed a "low risk" to the United States and could be contained, the position that Azar, Fauci, and Redfield maintained through most of February.

Navarro was not really trying to persuade them. He was aiming more at the president, to convince him to do the China travel ban. Trump, at that time, was emphasizing friendliness toward China's leader, with whom he had just signed a long-awaited trade deal.[12]

At this point, on January 28 and 29, lasting patterns of disagreement in the government were emerging. Despite such disagreements, we believe that on January 28 the U.S.

government should have started mobilizing for a possible Covid war, whatever it decided to do about a travel ban with China (which President Trump ordered a couple of days later).

President Trump and his advisers did not need to be sure that a pandemic was coming to the United States. Though it had not come from the intelligence community, America's leaders had received the equivalent of a strategic warning of possible imminent war.

It was hard for non-experts to grasp this. As far as they knew, no one had died yet from the virus in the United States.

The experts knew that, if this was a pandemic, every day counted. Naturally all could agree on trying to keep the outbreak out of the United States. Yet the risk of a pandemic was, at this point, great enough to at least put mobilization plans in motion.

As is often the case, experts disagreed. They did not have enough information from or in China. The warning intelligence did not come from traditional intelligence collection or formal reports. It relied on just the kinds of networks to gain added situation awareness that we called out in chapter 2.[13]

Some experts wanted to wait for more information. They relied on past experience to judge that the risk to the United States remained low or could likely be contained.

Others, from Farrar to Mecher to Borio to Pottinger, did not give the virus the benefit of the doubt. If the danger was even just a significant possibility, that should have been good enough to prompt a mobilization, weighing the costs of action against the potential costs of delay.

During the first weeks of February, when Azar was leading task force briefings in the White House press room with the "low risk to the United States" message, President Trump—joining that message in public—was privately telling reporter Bob Woodward (for instance on February 7) that "it goes through air, Bob, that's always tougher than the touch . . . You just breathe the air, that's how it's passed. So that's a very tricky one. . . . It's also more deadly than even your strenuous flus." But, on March 19, now in full public emergency mode, Trump explained to Woodward that "I wanted to always play it down. I still like playing it down, because I don't want to create a panic."

The panic was there without any presidential help. What was missing was the mobilization and readiness that would reassure the American people with action. In that same conversation, on March 19, Woodward channeled Trump's own advisors, impressing upon him the need for an aggressive strategy. "What's the plan now?" Woodward asked. "What are the next steps?"

"My next steps, Bob," Trump replied, "is I have to do a great job."[14]

What would it mean to start mobilizing for a Covid war? As we said at the end of the previous chapter, government readiness was not good. Available emergency money was minuscule. As we pointed out in the previous chapter, the president could have used Stafford Act authorities, used for domestic disaster relief, in order to release ample emergency funds. Those funds were held by FEMA, in the Department of Homeland Security. That money could have been used by HHS.

Also, some of what could, and should, have been done immediately was what Bright had already started planning and what Borio and Gottlieb had called for in the *Wall Street Journal*: starting up all engines for mass development, production, and deployment of tests, drugs, and vaccines, as well as personal protective equipment, like masks. They and others foresaw at the time that travel screening or quarantines might only be a first line of defense, good only until the virus started spreading inside the United States.

Beyond those points, we also wish to emphasize that ordering mass production was not enough. In chapter 1 we discussed three cultures of governance: cultures of programs/process, of research/investigation, and of operations. Mass production is not an operational strategy.

If there were an operational strategy for just how tests would be used, that strategy could then be coordinated with leadership at the FDA. The FDA could then tailor regulations on effectiveness of tests, for example, to the planned context of use and the need for rapid distribution across America. However, FDA commissioner Stephen Hahn was not even included in the task force for the first month.

Take testing, for example. If the production problems were being solved and a hundred thousand tests became available the next week, how would they have been used? To make a reliable diagnosis for treatment? To do a preliminary screen for possible illness with some simpler test? For biomedical surveillance? Who should be screened? How would the tests be deployed? Would the first priority be to distribute them to hospitals to create a biomedical surveillance system and track the enemy? Such a system had not been designed. Or would the priority be to distribute tests at drive-through locations for millions of panicked citizens? Should the tests be used to screen essential workers or keep schools open?

A real strategy would have to answer such questions, set clear purposes and priorities for which would be met first. It would take time to do this work well, so—in the absence of prior preparedness—an emergency effort had to begin right away. Such an effort would line up the needed people or firms, the organizations to manage them, and the money to pay them, on a nationwide scale. In other words, preparation is about much more than a stockpile of stuff in a warehouse.

By the end of January, as the World Health Organization officially declared a "public health emergency of international concern," most experts joined the general alarm. There were urgent questions, for instance about how to evacuate American citizens from Wuhan. The most important issues, though, were still about what to do.

CONTAINMENT POLICY DESIGNS

Innumerable speeches, books, and articles have stated that the Obama administration gave the incoming Trump administration a "playbook" on how to confront a pandemic and that this playbook was ignored. The Obama administration did indeed prepare and leave behind the "Playbook for Early Response to High-Consequence Emerging Infectious Disease Threats and Biological Incidents."[15]

But the playbook did not actually diagram any plays. There was no "how." It did not explain what to do.

Those who read that playbook will see that it was really a diagnostic manual. It provided sets of questions. As they worked through the questions, officials were supposed to determine whether a threat had moved up to being "elevated," then to "credible," and then to one or another stage of "public health emergency." Depending on the diagnosis, officials might invoke some special legal authority. Depending on the diagnosis, officials could consider "border screening" or dispatching disaster assistance teams.

But this last part, the "how" part, was never mapped out in the playbook. It did not outline just how to go about screening millions of incoming travelers. There was no description of just what, if there really were a truly global "high-consequence" event, the assistance teams were supposed to do.

The relevant officials in January 2020 had not ignored the so-called playbook. Many of them were career people. They knew the vocabulary for the various threat classifications and statutory authorities. But when it came to the job of how to contain a pandemic that was headed for the United States, in January 2020, the playbook was a blank page.

To operate on a significant scale, a pandemic containment had to

- have a plan—the "sheet music"—for roles and missions;
- regulate travel;
- screen potential cases; and
- quarantine and contact trace.

The CDC promptly activated its capacity to do all of these things on a small scale, including regulating travel out of China and screening incoming travelers. The screening was limited to people with symptoms of disease who had some relation to Wuhan. The system quickly started breaking down.

In the U.S. government, most of February 2020 was dominated by two themes. There was a hope to somehow keep the outbreak away from the United States with a fragmentary containment effort. And there were constant, consuming arguments micromanaging the repatriation of U.S. citizens from China or from cruise ships. The big muscle movements to mobilize U.S. preparedness for a pandemic were absent. Or, as one task force member put it: "In hindsight, we were focusing all of the task force on getting a kitty cat off the third floor, while the whole building was on fire and there were a thousand people in it."[16]

At the very least, before addressing the demand for caregiving, drugs, or vaccines, the United States had to build a screening system and a strategy for how to use whatever tests it could deploy. Brett Giroir, then the assistant secretary for health at HHS, oversaw the Public Health Service. Giroir acknowledged that "we were the deployable health care force," but it was "understaffed and undertrained historically." Also, he acknowledged, as did Redfield, that officials were influenced by an "influenza" model in which infected people displayed clear symptoms and little testing was needed.[17]

"I'd been very involved with the [2014] Ebola outbreak in Texas," Giroir later recalled. "So you have to test, you know, 50 people, right? Influenza—you don't need testing. It was just not part of any plan here. I don't think there had been, in any administration, true discussions with the industry about what a public-private partnership [for mass production of testing] would look like."[18]

In other countries, though, those mass plans and industry discussions were in place. Few large countries with a lot of international travel did well in keeping the virus out of their country. The ones that did best were islands with few ports of entry. One of the outstanding success stories for containment was South Korea.

South Korea is, functionally, akin to an island because its border with North Korea is so tightly closed. But it is a densely populated country of more than 50 million people and with a large number of international travelers—more than 17 million incoming and outgoing during the year before the pandemic. It is a noisy democracy with power nearly equally balanced between bitterly divided rival political parties.

Jolted by miscues during the SARS epidemic of 2002–04 and the MERS outbreak of 2012–14, the South Korean government had evaluated its mistakes. In 2015, Korea passed new laws and made its CDC a powerful independent agency with broad authorities and regional centers, charged to do better next time. The government developed policy designs for what to do. Knowing that even the new agency could not do these things on its own, its evolving policy design identified private firms, medical services, and resources for local health workers.

Another notable success story in containment was Germany. Germany has a population about one-fourth the size of the United States. Like the United States, Germany has a federal system, and executive decisions about public health are mainly made in the health departments of its sixteen states (*Länder*) and hundreds of counties. Germany also has strong laws to protect patient and data privacy. German public health uses a federal research entity, the Robert Koch Institute, as a central player in its national response.

Like South Korea, Germany entered the crisis with a "national pandemic plan." Though the Robert Koch Institute did not control the state and local health departments, there were very strong common standards in training and standardization of methods.

When the Covid invasion began, big countries with a lot of travelers had very little time to figure out how to keep the pandemic away from their shores. By mid-March 2020, as the scale of the pandemic was becoming obvious to everyone, the opportunity to contain it was already gone, unless a working policy was already in business.

Germany's challenge, with its extensive land borders and intra-European travel, was especially great. Countries like South Korea and the United States had more of a chance to screen incoming travelers from Asia and Europe.

On the surface, South Korean, German, and American policies might seem similar. Each started screening travel from Wuhan and from China at about the same time. Each were checking for symptoms.

But the Koreans and Germans had a defined policy design for screening that involved a lot of testing (tens of thousands a day by mid-February), quick (same-day) results from a growing network of prepared labs, quarantine procedures and facilities for positive cases, and case workers to assist people who were told to self-quarantine.

In the United States, the American CDC, which had the lead for proposing containment policies, had many of the same ideas. The Americans also had the capacity and resources, in theory, to do everything the Koreans and Germans did, and do it on the proportionately greater scale. Germany, for instance, spends *much* less on healthcare, as a proportion of GDP, than the United States does (about 12 percent versus about 20 percent).[19]

Hence, a crucial difference, from the start, was that both the Koreans and Germans, two other democracies, had developed quite comprehensive plans for national biomedical surveillance of every suspect case in practically every health facility, with data sharing anonymized to protect privacy, and paired with personal follow-up. The United States had not.

Later, the state of the art evolved to include rapid genomic sequencing. The British and the South Africans were some of the best performers. The British could even link genomic testing with clinical surveillance. Again, the United States would lag.

A big part of the problem was the weak infrastructure to do this work in America. Yet the Americans also did not have what we have called the "software," the software of planning, policy design, organization, and practice. Software design embeds an architecture of programmed steps and alternatives, laboriously tested and improved. One of America's more consistently effective public servants, James

Baker, had a family maxim he called his "five P's": "Prior Preparation Prevents Poor Performance."

As February 2020 went on, it became obvious that the CDC, and the government as a whole, did not have a well-developed policy design to carry out appropriate screening operations in the less than twenty international gateways that handled almost all of the air travelers entering or exiting the United States.

- There was not a design for whole-of-government cooperation.

- The CDC did not have the authority or plans to utilize other medical institutions and call up the state and local health departments, which themselves had little ability to mount large testing operations.

- It had almost no workable Covid tests throughout the month of February. Indeed, relatively few tests were available even during the month of March.

- It had almost no capacity to get same-day results even on the tests it did have, in part because it did not have a reliable network of supporting labs.

The CDC's quarantine facilities (though a traditional part of its mission) turned out, in practice, to be practically useless for large-scale Covid quarantines. The CDC had to do some frantic work with the Pentagon just to figure out ways to hold American citizens repatriated from Wuhan on military bases and quarantine some cruise passengers taken off infected ships.

SILENT SPREAD AND THE ABSENCE OF
BIOMEDICAL SURVEILLANCE

Because of these policy design problems, the American containment strategy stalled after the initial start at screening and limiting travel from China. Soon, by early February 2020, cases were also flowing into the United States from Europe, mostly undetected. For months, influenced by habits of thinking about influenza, the CDC also tended to concentrate its attention on symptomatic spread. It therefore could not design a containment strategy that could pick up and track most of the entering cases.

In those early weeks, although the number of known cases seemed very small, the CDC's and others' attention to banning travel was an increasingly futile way of coping with the inability to screen, or even identify, suspect travelers. American leaders faced a seemingly binary choice between either doing a travel ban—for instance on travelers coming from Europe—or doing nothing. On February 11, Redfield asked President Trump to stop incoming travel from Europe.[20]

This sort of choice, the resort to blunt instruments because no better ones were available, was an ominous sign of things to come. Subsequent evidence has confirmed that, after the first week of February, travel bans would probably have been useless. The virus was already in the country and cases were being generated locally much faster than they could be imported into the United States.[21]

When there was so little testing going on, and cases were already being confirmed, the leaders could have inferred that the value of border screening was fading. The enemy had already broken through the first line of defense. It was time to focus on domestic health surveillance and "mitigation"—community defense.

Outside of the health agencies, officials were understandably shocked at proposals for wholesale travel bans. Until mid-March 2020, they opposed them. One reaction among such officials, then, was to downplay the problem. President Trump kept telling citizens that everything was fine, that the United States was in no danger. Just the opposite was true.

But hesitation about travel bans was typical everywhere. Even in South Korea, the special processing requirements were implemented in different areas gradually, without jumping to general bans. In the United States, this hesitation meant that, for travelers who were not coming from China, there were no bans and little screening at all.

Instead of travel bans, the U.S. government needed a national strategy for biomedical surveillance. Such a strategy would be designed to track the progress and character of the enemy, to inform the many defense choices that were coming. Such surveillance can drive the assessments in forecasts and modeling, providing information about the genetic variants in circulation, their per-case severity, and the effectiveness of drugs and vaccines.

To track when and where the virus was making its way into the United States, until the beginning of March the CDC relied on voluntary reporting of confirmed Covid cases from hospitals or from state or local health departments. While continuing its usual surveillance of reported influenza-like illnesses and emergency respiratory cases, on March 1, the CDC adapted its existing hospital surveillance network to add careful tracking of Covid cases.

This COVID-NET helped with real-time research. But it was not a comprehensive aid to biomedical surveillance. Its fourteen participating geographic areas covered about 10 percent of the U.S. population. It could not help with contact tracing in any practical way.[22]

No federal agency, including the CDC, had designed or tried to build a rapid-action, interdisciplinary, systematic biomedical surveillance network. Such a network would show how many people were getting sick, reveal what kind of people were most vulnerable and the key risk factors, illustrate the usual course of the disease, and employ robust capabilities for genomic sequencing.

The federal government had invested (through Anthony Fauci's part of NIH) nearly a billion dollars since 2003 for a national network of regional and national biocontainment labs. These labs were supposed to address dangers from emerging infectious diseases or bioterrorism but these were dedicated to basic research, not biomedical surveillance.[23]

At the end of March, the CDC, desperate to create some method of real-time biomedical surveillance, asked tech firms for help. Apple and Google released an app for their iOS and Android platforms so that people could report their Covid status in their states. But, even then, public health authorities had neither the power nor the staff to link this app to a system for monitoring people in self-quarantine or follow up with case workers.[24]

When Deborah Birx became the coordinator of the White House Coronavirus Task Force, she found herself

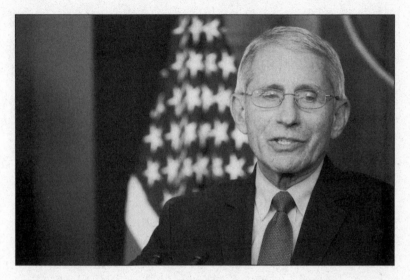

Anthony Fauci, Director of the National Institute of Allergy and Infectious Diseases, speaking at the White House Coronavirus Task Force press briefing on April 22, 2020. PHOTO CREDIT: MANDEL NGAN/ AFP VIA GETTY IMAGES

relying for information on a data tracking system set up by an engineering professor at Johns Hopkins University. Breaking down data by U.S. states and territories, the Covid Tracking Project organized by a team at *Atlantic* magazine was also more useful in real time than the CDC's surveillance efforts.[25]

Therefore, policies were being designed largely in the dark, reacting as people showed up in hospitals, sick and dying. In 2021, when the Biden administration took office, the U.S. government still had not created such a network.

Therefore, in 2021, the CDC and the U.S. government again failed to adequately assess an incoming viral invasion. This time it was the invasion of the COVID-19 Delta variant that took so many lives later that year, followed by the Omicron wave, which took still more. This continued weakness in surveillance led to the Biden administration's crisis managers being caught off-balance as they were paring back investments in tests and drugs.

Some other countries did have better biomedical surveillance. Throughout the war, U.S. experts constantly ended up having to rely on assessments from those countries that did collect the data and do the analysis for good biomedical intelligence work. These were countries like Israel, Denmark, and the United Kingdom, and later, South Africa.

Good systems to collect such data in real time and put it to use had already been up and running in Britain, building on the data routinely collected in its National Health Service. Though its healthcare system is different, the United States could build on foundations both in government (the giant Centers for Medicare and Medicaid Services, CMS) and the big healthcare companies. Early in 2020, British researchers and officials mapped out how to use their system to get the Covid information they might need. Britain later established the UK Health Security Agency to consolidate the old Public Health England with other testing and biodefense agencies. The British experts figured out how to access needed data while protecting patient privacy.

In 2021, the new Biden administration created the Center for Forecasting and Outbreak Analytics (CFA). They put it in the CDC. It started with a small staff, recruiting one of us to help. It is a small office facing an overwhelming need.

In the winter of 2021–22, as a proof of concept, the CFA worked with Kaiser Permanente–Southern California to set up an Israel-style data collection system in order to help evaluate the new Omicron wave of Covid then arriving in the United States. The stars were in alignment for this pilot project—the right people and data agreements were already in place.[26]

The project worked. It provided insightful information in just a few weeks. This can be done here. But CFA's experiment occurred two years into the pandemic.

THE TESTING PROBLEM BEGINS

Even if the CDC had recognized and spotlighted the danger of asymptomatic—silent—spread, it would have had trouble implementing any biomedical surveillance strategy unless the U.S. government could have deployed many thousands of tests. In that first month or two, in the containment stage, the need for tests was large, but manageable. Tens of thousands were needed, not yet tens of millions.[27]

The first Covid tests were PCR (polymerase chain reaction) tests that test for the presence of the virus, or fragments of it. They require laboratory processing. By the summer of 2020, antigen tests, which detect the presence of viral protein, were becoming available. These tests are easier to administer and process. Each kind has strengths and weaknesses. PCR tests tend to produce more false positives, detecting the remnants of a departed virus. Antigen tests definitely show a virus is present if they are positive, but they might miss the beginning of an infection, so they have more false negatives early in the onset of the disease.

The American problems with developing and distributing good Covid tests became notorious. What went wrong in this stage, when PCR tests, with their lab processing, were what was available?

- The CDC did a good, quick job of developing a Covid test, but made avoidable errors in the test design and scaling up production.

- The CDC relied on its network of state public health labs to use the test and process results, an approach that could not scale to mass needs.

- Until the end of February, the FDA banned anyone but CDC, such as the hundreds of academic and hospital labs, from developing and using a Covid test unless they first went through a cumbersome process to get an FDA "emergency use authorization."

- The U.S. government did not begin engaging private industry, and its high-volume processing network of labs, to tackle this problem on a mass scale until the crisis was well underway.

The FDA issue needs a closer look. The FDA had a legitimate interest in making sure that people did not peddle worthless tests to an anxious public. The problem was more one of coordinated strategy. If the purpose of the test was well defined, either for highly reliable diagnosis or just as a more limited screening tool, that could set a standard for test design. The FDA might then, playing its part in a government-wide strategy, proactively encourage and help many producers make what was needed—or import them from friendly countries.

With virus samples in hand, the real challenge in producing diagnostic tests is not scientific. The challenge is scaling the logistics of mass, high-quality production, then doing distribution at affordable cost, and then developing an ordering and reporting system to get quick test results from a parallel network of certified labs.

Again, the contrasts with South Korea and Germany offer some insight. South Korea knew, ahead of time, that it would have to rely on private firms to meet that challenge. Before the Covid war, candidate firms had already been recruited for this mission and given some money to prepare. During January, the Korean CDC (the Korea Disease Control and Prevention Agency, or KDCA) started preparing a test for any coronaviruses. As soon as it got virus samples, the KDCA called in its private partners. On January 27, the KDCA was sharing everything with the private firms and committing to large advance purchases of the tests they would produce, if the firms met the KDCA's specifications. In other words, the KDCA already had its own kind of Operation Warp Speed, for testing, in place by the end of January. That is why, by mid-February, South Korea could run tens of thousands of tests a day. At that moment, the U.S. conversations with industry were only beginning.

Germany was one of the first countries in the world to develop a reliable COVID-19 test. It did this in January. Its test was quickly adopted as the standard by the World Health Organization. Providers and state governments in the United States could not import or use it because it was not authorized by the FDA.

Germany shared necessary information with private firms. The Germans immediately clarified how such testing would be paid for, in both their public and private health insurance systems. The operation of such payment systems was well understood. It was clear the government would be using testing on a massive scale. Thus, Germany's major private firms, like Bosch, could confidently ramp up large-scale production and distribution.

The CDC and the FDA tried, at first, to limit who would be tested unless there was some clinical reason for it, such as if that person was symptomatic and had a recent travel connection to China. The CDC did not change that guidance until February 29.

In the meantime, the FDA invoked a provision that prohibited the use of laboratory-developed tests (LDTs) once the public health emergency was declared. The FDA is more decentralized than it may seem to outsiders. Key decisions really devolve to its specialized "centers": one for drugs (headed in 2020 by Janet Woodcock), one for vaccines/biologics (headed in 2020 by Peter Marks), and one for devices and radiology. This last is the Center for Devices and Radiological Health, headed in 2020 by Jeffrey Shuren. The office in the center that handled tests was headed by Tim Stenzel.

LDTs are tests developed and employed in certified, highly competent laboratories. They are common in large hospital and academic clinical labs. The move by the FDA's devices center restricted all clinical testing to the flawed CDC test and the few other tests that worked their costly way through the Emergency Use Authorization process.

The American approach was then, belatedly, to urge the large existing test producers in the private sector, like Roche, Thermo Fisher, and Abbott, to start producing tests at scale. Some of these companies had actually produced tests during the SARS crisis of 2002–04 and then been burned when the market for this work evaporated.

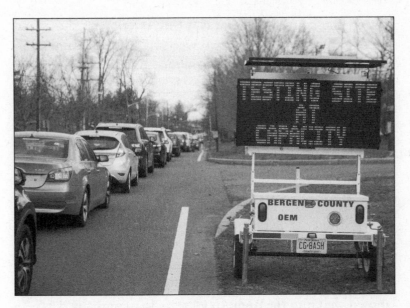

Cars lining up for drive-through Covid testing at a facility at
Bergen Community College in Paramus, New Jersey, on March 21,
2020. PHOTO CREDIT: ANGUS MORDANT/BLOOMBERG VIA GETTY IMAGES

Until at least March and April 2020, the federal government did not have a plan to subsidize test development and
deployment and production at scale, with its own requirements then driving the process. Even once Covid tests were
on the market, it took weeks or months for pharmacies and
other point-of-care testing locations to get the necessary
waivers and reimbursement structures in place to perform
tests in their communities.

Only a few days after it began easing the rules on test production and use, on March 3, the CDC reported that it
could confirm that the United States already had at least
sixty cases of COVID-19 in twelve different states, scattered

around the country. This was a tiny fraction of the actual number. During the next two weeks, President Trump and other world leaders would announce national emergencies and nationwide lockdowns.

On March 11, the president's son-in-law, Jared Kushner, became a central figure in managing the crisis. He intervened to help settle a raging argument about banning travel from Europe (they banned it). He then drafted a speech the president gave that night from the Oval Office to announce this ban, a speech that had not gone well.

On March 12, Kushner tried to break the testing bottleneck. He joined prolonged task force discussions about how to engage leaders from the private sector in distributing and deploying tests. The White House Coronavirus Task Force labored well into the night to identify key company partners and the roles they could play.

Kushner called company executives and urged them to come to Washington the next day, March 13, for a meeting with the president and a public announcement in the Rose Garden. At last, the administration would announce a warlike mobilization. Flanked by the executives, President Trump announced that there would be testing sites at Walgreens and CVS drugstores all over America. Google would build a website that would digest people's symptoms, determine if they needed a test, and tell them where to go.

It took only hours for journalists and the public to realize that the mobilization was, at best, a hastily invented set of hopes, if it was not—more cynically—just smoke and mirrors. There were no such sites at CVS or Walgreens stores and the local officials who were supposed to staff them had not heard of the plan. There were not enough tests to provide even if the sites were ready. The supplies to manufacture such tests had not been nailed down. Google had no such website, though an affiliated company, Verily (formerly Google Life Sciences), timorously promised that the website was "in the early stages of development."[28]

These three issues—the problems of overall policy design, the misjudgment about silent spread combined with weakness of biomedical surveillance, and the limited availability of tests—all played out in the next stage of the Covid war. In the next stage, every community in America would struggle to defend itself.

5

FEDERAL CRISIS MANAGEMENT COLLAPSES; OPERATION WARP SPEED BEGINS

A YEAR BEFORE THE pandemic, during the first months of 2019, the ASPR office in HHS, led by Robert Kadlec, ran a set of exercises to test readiness for a pandemic. The exercises—there were four of them between January and May—assumed that a new influenza virus (H7N9) had arrived in the United States, coming out of China. This flu was assumed to have an infection fatality rate of about half of one percent (a number not that far off from the eventual rate for COVID-19).

The ASPR's job in these exercises was to mitigate the virus impact and help communities defend themselves. The ASPR would practice how to organize medical countermeasures to fight back.

Most books about the Covid crisis mention this exercise. It was called Crimson Contagion. They note that the exercise revealed coordination problems with the authorities who would have to respond in the field, the Federal Emergency Management Agency over at the Department of Homeland Security and the state and local authorities. In the exercise, hosted in Chicago, participants argued about issues that came up, like orders to close schools. The exercise also helped Kadlec and his aides realize that his office did not have enough money to order up new vaccines. In the exercise, hundreds of thousands died.

What the books do not mention about this exercise is that two of its basic premises turned out to be poor guides for the Covid war. The Crimson Contagion exercise, like much of the government's pandemic planning, assumed that the outbreak would be from a kind of influenza. With influenza, symptoms usually appear soon after a person becomes able to transmit infection, so there is less reliance on tests to spot people who are infected and a risk to others.

The exercise thus did not spotlight a key feature of the coronavirus pandemic, asymptomatic transmission. That meant the exercise also did not spotlight how important it would be to scale up the mass production of tests, lab capacity to process them, and the means to finance and deploy them.

More important: The Crimson Contagion exercise assumed that the government had medicine to treat this hypothetical flu. The exercise assumed there were at least 30 million doses on hand. The lockdowns and school closures in the exercise were therefore just meant to be temporary, to buy a little time, until this medicine could be distributed and healthcare delivery readied, while work on a vaccine was put in motion.[1]

In the Covid war, there were no such medicines at hand. The temporary lockdown and closures quickly and foreseeably spawned the question: If good medicines are not yet available, what should we do now?

EARLY SETUPS TO MANAGE THE CRISIS

In the first weeks of the crisis, the CDC was the incident manager. Once the potential scale became evident near the end of January, the White House created the Coronavirus Task Force. The HHS secretary, Alex Azar, became its chair. It was coordinated through the National Security Council system, in which Pottinger, the senior staffer who had sounded the alarm on January 28, played a large role.

This structure lasted through the month of February 2020, until the failure of containment. This was the period of constant preoccupation with travel restrictions at airports and repatriation of Americans back home, including stranded cruise ship passengers, while wider emergency mobilization efforts languished. It was a period of growing tension between CDC's role as incident manager and the simultaneous role of Kadlec, the ASPR, to organize a wider response. Everyone involved admits there was confusion and friction about who was in charge of what problems. The FDA was left out altogether, until being added in on March 1, on the insistence of the White House domestic policy chief Joe Grogan.

Kadlec's team reached out to FEMA early in February, knowing they might need the operational help, referring to a 2018 "Pandemic Crisis Action Plan." FEMA began assigning a few capable operators to HHS and readying scores of possible assistance teams. HHS and FEMA updated their Pandemic Crisis Action Plan, called PanCAP.[2]

This updated PanCAP, from March 2020, was not really an action plan. It was a jargon laden catalog of problems, diagrams of coordinating processes, and statements of goals. It was a programs/process document, not operational. There was little in it about what people would actually do, how they were to accomplish the tasks, or about priorities, sequencing, or costs.

For example, someone interested in the testing strategy might find mention of testing in a table of "lines of effort." There one could find a list of "intermediate objectives & tasks." Medical countermeasures were one of the lines of effort. The relevant statement just said: "Develop and distribute rapid diagnostic tests." The rest, hopefully, would be in other plans.[3]

Trained as a lawyer, HHS secretary Alex Azar was an experienced public official, very much in the programs/process mode. He had held top jobs in both the HHS department and in the private sector, leading the pharma company Eli Lilly. He listened to and tried to sift the views of the head of the CDC, Robert Redfield (who was splitting his time between Washington and Atlanta); the NIH leaders, Francis Collins and Anthony Fauci; and Kadlec.

On February 24, President Trump, traveling in India, tweeted: "The Coronavirus is very much under control in the USA. . . . Stock market starting to look very good to me!"[4]

That same day, Azar's task force agreed that containment was failing. They agreed it was time to prepare the United States for the traumatic transition to mitigation and community defense. Redfield relayed this decision to one of his key deputies, Nancy Messonnier.

In her press briefing the next morning, February 25, Messonnier announced: "We expect we will see community spread in this country. It's not so much a question of if this will happen anymore, but rather more a question of exactly when this will happen and how many people in this country will have severe illness." The stock market dived.[5]

President Trump was furious. He kept downplaying the danger. "It's going to disappear," he said on February 27. "Everything is really under control," he said on February 29. His top press and political aides continued to parrot this line on through the first week of March.[6]

In the furor after this episode, Azar began rearranging the Coronavirus Task Force. He made Kadlec the incident manager. He brought Giroir, the assistant secretary for health who looked after the Public Health Service, into the Task Force to be Kadlec's deputy. Giroir was soon asked to take charge of the testing problem, as a national coordinator authorized to tackle these issues with private industry, the FDA, and the CDC.

The testing problem had already grown well beyond the use of testing for containment. Now the government was under great pressure to make tests available to millions of worried Americans, perhaps through thousands of to-be-created "drive-through" testing sites.

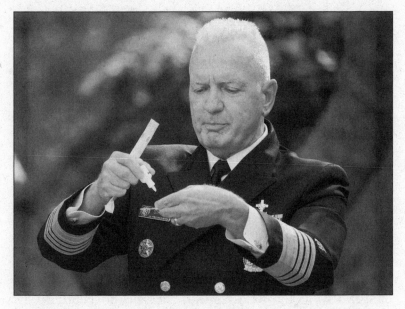

Brett Giroir, Assistant Secretary for Health and federal Covid testing czar, demonstrates using a self-test kit as he speaks in the White House Rose Garden on September 28, 2020. PHOTO CREDIT: MANDEL NGAN/AFP VIA GETTY IMAGES

One of Giroir's first issues was to try to develop tests that could just use shallow nasal swabs, that people could easily perform, swabbing their nose. The existing tests relied on elongated swabs, unfamiliar to most people, carefully inserted through the nose to get to the upper part of the throat behind the nose (the nasopharyngeal area). Such tests could only be performed by trained people, equipped with scarce personal protective equipment.

As Azar was rearranging these responsibilities, the White House planned to rearrange Azar's role. Grogan wanted to replace Azar with the former FDA head, Scott Gottlieb. The counterargument was that this move would lead Azar to resign, which might look bad. Finally the president and White House acting chief of staff Mulvaney solved the problem by asking Vice President Mike Pence to chair the task force. That, with some manhandling by Pence's chief of staff, Marc Short, would also allow the White House to, as one of Pence's staffers later put it, "make sure they had full control of the messaging" about the response.[7]

The White House, including President Trump's influential son-in-law, Jared Kushner, blamed Azar and Kadlec's office for the testing snafu and growing shortages of supplies. Kushner joined Giroir in directly reaching out to leaders of private industry to help. This was when Grogan brought the FDA's new leader, Stephen Hahn, into the task force.

The lead NSC staffer, Pottinger helped recruit a public health official managing a major health program in Africa, Deborah Birx, to come back to DC and become the task force's coordinator. Birx shared the general frustration with the CDC: "I was all about now-now-now action; they were all about 'wait for irrefutable data.'"[8]

Thus the new situation, in the first week of March 2020, was that Vice President Pence was in charge of federal crisis management, aided by Birx. But, because the vice president was in charge, the coordination was moved out of the National Security Council system and Pottinger's role declined. Since Pottinger had been Birx's principal sponsor, she became more isolated.

Azar's involvement in the response declined too, but he helped push for Kadlec to take charge of the pandemic response within HHS. That announcement went out on March 2. Yet, at the same time, Pence's staff kicked Kadlec out of the White House Task Force! "I got kind of voted off the island," Kadlec said, with a Pence staffer recalling that Kadlec had been "very vocal" about issues like depletion of the Strategic National Stockpile of needed equipment. The CDC's Redfield remained.[9]

Veterans of crisis management, whether they are domestic first responders or in the military, understand the value of going into an emergency with people who know each other and have some familiar routines, usually from prior practice. This wasn't the case in early March 2020. Most of these people had no experience working together under pressure, and this crisis management setup would only last for a couple of weeks.

THE COLLAPSE OF FEDERAL CRISIS MANAGEMENT

On March 13, 2020, President Trump could no longer deny the scale of the crisis. He, like other world leaders, declared a national emergency. This invoked the Stafford Act and finally released FEMA's disaster relief funds to help address the crisis. States were entitled to ask for help. The FEMA administrator, Peter Gaynor, began passing authority to his regional administrators because "it's never happened that every region has entered a disaster at once . . . this was the biggest thing FEMA has seen." Following the advice of the Pence-led task force, this emergency included a broad national lockdown and curtailment of travel meant to last for a short time: "15 Days to Slow the Spread."[10]

This move was followed, later in March, by a $2.3 trillion economic stimulus package, the Coronavirus Aid, Relief, and Economic Security (CARES) Act. There was little planning behind it. Rather than start figuring out how to adapt businesses and employment to the pandemic, the plan simply gave out stunning sums of money to the American people. Economists sometimes refer to such blanket stimulus as "helicopter money," since the theory is not far from the idea of just throwing money out of a helicopter flying over a city. This was the largest helicopter money experiment in the history of the United States. In his memoir, Kushner simply wrote: "We were shooting bullets into a cloud of smoke and hoping that enough of them would hit their targets to save an economy veering toward collapse."[11]

During those "15 Days to Slow the Spread," as the country was alarmed by news of crowded emergency rooms—and morgues—in Italy and then New York City, the White House reevaluated how it wished to handle this crisis. Part of the early March White House reorganization included a new chief of staff to the president (his fourth). Mulvaney was out. Grogan soon followed him out the door. The new chief of staff was a North Carolina congressman, Mark Meadows.

As the crisis escalated, connected officials and business leaders began bypassing the Pence-led task force and went directly to Kushner for help. As we mentioned in the previous chapter, by March 12, Kushner, who was a kind of White House chief of staff on the issues he worked on, had started taking over the problem of organizing private industry to get supplies and solve the testing problem, which at that time was dominated less by a coherent medical or economic strategy than by a rush to set up drive-through sites to serve justifiably fearful citizens.

With the emergency declaration, another set of federal procedures clicked in that brought the Federal Emergency Management Agency into the foreground. On March 18, President Trump told FEMA leader Gaynor to "take over." With FEMA's involvement came another interagency structure for coordinating a national response with 24/7 links around the country. But FEMA was an instrument, not a source of guidance. It was used to being in a support role.

Hearing of President Trump's guidance, one of FEMA's key operators began whiteboarding what to do, which he called a "surreal experience reorganizing the government in two hours." FEMA had operational experience and ability, but no public health strategy for how best to track and fight the pandemic. Knowing this, its leaders roped in HHS, including Kadlec and his team, and someone from CDC, to help guide decisions. In other words, FEMA had capability but a murky picture of what to do, except rush toward whatever was the problem du jour (e.g., urgent calls from this or that place for PPE, a push to set up drive-through test sites). FEMA was also tasked to help Kushner's ad hoc efforts.[12]

It is worth pausing briefly to note how the federal crisis management had splintered by the third week of March. There was still the Pence-chaired task force. There was Kushner taking increasing charge of his plans to handle supplies (Kadlec's nominal job). There was FEMA and Gaynor, told they were in charge. There were the various HHS entities— CDC, NIH, ASPR, FDA—trying to fit in somehow while, at HHS, Giroir was the new "testing czar."

During this same period, late-March to late-April, the White House came very close to just firing Azar—a "razor's edge," one participant in the discussions told us. Instead, the White House, with Kushner and Meadows on point, decided it was best to keep him, after Azar was told to shape up, in a direct discussion with one of Kushner's friends. Meadows and Kushner, and presumably President Trump, seemed to have thought Azar would be more pliable than any likely alternative.[13]

All these organizational efforts found themselves jammed by the consequences of earlier decisions that gave Kadlec and ASPR very little money to implement emergency strategies, even if the strategies had been good ones. For instance, as we mentioned earlier, loud calls—including constructive ideas from industry—for a crash program to buy N95 masks had been circulating in Kadlec's office since the third week of January. Kadlec had no money, no real emergency fund. The Trump administration first went to Congress with a supplemental funding request of $1.25 billion in new money on February 24, and money did not start to flow until March. BARDA head Rick Bright recalled that "OMB played with us for weeks. . . . You cannot plan a big response by nickel and diming."[14]

The combination of Meadows and Kushner began providing fresh direction on how President Trump would tackle the spreading pandemic. Their approach had three aspects, not necessarily in harmony.

First, Kushner and his aides, based at FEMA or the White House, created an emergency effort to supplement what they regarded as a feeble effort by Azar and Kadlec to meet the urgent demand for supplies such as PPE and ventilators. Working with FEMA they also created a program called Project Airbridge. FEMA would help fly supplies to where they were needed. Kushner and his aides reached out to private executives to get needed supplies of many kinds, which would then presumably be routed out to those who needed them, using FEMA's help. They hoped to use the Defense Production Act (DPA) to help commandeer materials. President Trump signed an executive order, in May, granting one of these aides, Adam Boehler, powers to use the DPA and some money.[15]

This emergency program, based out of FEMA and its National Response Coordination Center, lasted for only three months. It wound up its work in June 2020. It plainly offered some help. The value of that help can be weighed against the added confusion this parallel effort brought to the already stressed system, as many officials began going directly to Kushner to get what they needed. The help did not make a fundamental impact on the availability of needed supplies. It is hard to tell just what this effort was able to accomplish in the spring and summer of 2020.

Second, and much more fundamental than Kushner's stopgap measures, President Trump, Meadows, and Kushner appear to have decided that the strategic-level governance of how to manage the public health crisis, and the political responsibility and accountability for that, would move out of the federal government. The public health management would go down to the states and cities.

On Saturday evening, March 21, Kushner met in the White House Situation Room with a group of private CEOs, who expected to hear the outlines of the broad government plan to buy supplies, using the DPA, and deploy them where needed most. Kushner told them: "The federal government is not going to lead this response. It's up to the states to figure out what they want to do." In June 2020, the FEMA-HHS "realigned" from "take charge" into working groups that would just support the state, tribal, and territorial crisis management efforts.[16]

Third, President Trump, Meadows, and others at the White House decided that the experts were exaggerating the seriousness of the public health problem. President Trump had already been taken with the idea that the Covid outbreak was no worse than a bad flu season. For a short time he had seemed to back off of that belief. By early April he was back there again. Economic analysts at the White House were developing their own critiques of the health data. They reached out to sympathetic healthcare pundits, like Scott Atlas. At this time Atlas believed the American death toll from the pandemic might be about ten thousand. The White House later recruited Atlas to join the White House staff as an adviser on the crisis.[17]

During the late spring of 2020, this bubble of optimism about the crisis became an important part of the story. The bubble started deflating by June, when a second wave started sweeping the country (though it was really just the widening ripples from the first wave of the viral spread). That bubble was decisively dispelled in the late autumn and winter of 2020–21 by the real second wave of the pandemic, which for the United States was the deadliest single phase of the war.

These last two aspects of the White House choice, to diminish the federal role and downplay the seriousness of the crisis, were obviously connected. By early April, deep into his reelection campaign, President Trump had become convinced that the country had to reopen for the economy to improve. Responsibility for unpopular public health measures would move out of the White House. And the only way to defend this approach was to hope, or presume, that the problem was not that serious.

The net effect of the White House abandonment of federal crisis management in March and April 2020 was that the new interagency machinery, the White House task force supposedly being run by Vice President Pence and the newly recruited coordinator, Birx, became even more disconnected from what was going on.

On March 31, Birx helped persuade President Trump to endorse a thirty-day extension of lockdowns to "slow the spread." Later that week, on April 3, the President turned angrily on Birx, in the narrow hallway connecting the West Wing to the White House Briefing Room. "We will never shut down the country again. Never." The president acted as if Birx had betrayed him.[18]

Birx soon realized, early in April, that her month-old relationship with President Trump was irretrievably torn. She learned that some of the president's economic staff had assured the president that Birx's estimates of the public health danger were greatly exaggerated and that, by Memorial Day, the United States might suffer only about 26,000 deaths (Birx's staff had predicted about 100,000 to 240,000). This lower estimate tended to reinforce the "it's like flu" argument.

That economic staff estimate was wrong. As of April 8, there were already at least eighteen thousand deaths and the numbers were rising by more than two thousand a day. Birx "suspected then, and am now absolutely convinced, that by the time I got [a copy of the economic staff estimate], I had already been many days behind in the race for the president's attention and trust. I am sure that in every internal senior

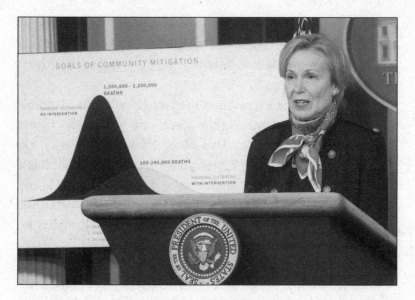

White House coronavirus response coordinator Deborah Birx speaks during the daily coronavirus task force briefing at the White House on March 31, 2020. In the background is a graphic representing projected Covid deaths with and without mitigation measures. PHOTO CREDIT: WIN MCNAMEE/GETTY IMAGES

advisor discussion, the president was reminded of just how wrong I had been in my projections. It never mattered that my projections were right then and continued to be right throughout 2020 and 2021; being right apparently didn't matter."

As April went on, Birx also realized that much of the White House was actually becoming an adversary in her efforts. "If April was when the economic forces in the White House regrouped against the science of the virus, May saw us increasingly marginalized, solidifying President Trump's, and his administration's, resistance to our efforts. As the tide turned, the mood grew darker, more sinister." This ominous climate manifested itself, for example, in repeated threats against Birx and her family, as well as frequent threats against Anthony Fauci.

President Trump remained interested, though, in dominating the national messaging about the crisis, which was gripping public attention. This lasted a few more weeks. He made regular television appearances in the White House pressroom to talk about the crisis and what he was doing, usually with Birx or Fauci standing uncomfortably off to the side. On March 24, he told a Fox News interviewer that he "would love to have the country opened up and just raring to go by Easter [April 12]." But later that day, in the pressroom, Trump was more careful and deferential to the experts.[19]

By late April, as a frightened and bewildered country became more and more confused about continuing business and school closures, and after some brow-raising comments at a White House briefing in which he discussed treating the virus with light, heat, or disinfectant, Trump essentially detached himself from his own government. He moved toward questioning and challenging what other government officials were doing.

Presidents usually lead in times of crisis in order to help address the fears of fellow Americans. Trump was asked in a White House briefing how he would calm Americans' fears. He dismissed the question as "nasty." That answer prompted one group, "The Call to Unite," to enlist a former president (George W. Bush) to record a widely covered message to the American people.[20]

From the top, with President Trump, the administration had no real will to offer federal executive direction to the field, to offset weaknesses of the outdated American public health structure. The administration abdicated its wartime responsibility to lead. It left the battlefield, and the war strategy, to state militias (led by their governors) and ad hocism at the local level.

Even if the administration had chosen to offer federal executive direction, it would have been difficult to do it, given the outdated health structure and the policy failures that left the country so unprepared when the pandemic hit. We discussed those in chapter 3, "The Defenders." But it was not too late to build up biomedical surveillance and develop more effective national strategies.

That did not happen. The White House was more and more distanced from the daily management of the crisis. In April, Meadows regarded the Pence-Birx task force as "useless and broken."[21]

The final symptom of the policymaking void was the reliance for leadership, among the insiders, on people like Kushner. Or, among those on the outside, there was Anthony Fauci, an official who was not in a policy job, but who instead directed an institution that sponsored and evaluated scientific research. Fauci and his boss, NIH head Francis Collins, did have a critical role to play, but it was more in the realm of evaluating medical countermeasures, not the management of a public health crisis.

But Fauci had played a part advising on medical crises for six previous presidents. In a situation without any really coherent policymaking apparatus, people looked to Fauci so desperately because he seemed like the only adult in the room. He did speak more truthfully about the seriousness of the pandemic. Fauci, unlike Azar, had his own connections to the press. Unable to muzzle Fauci, the Trump White House and its supporters began attacking him. Fauci was vulnerable to some attacks because he tried to cover the waterfront in briefing the press and public, stretching beyond his core expertise—and sometimes it showed.

THE CREATION OF
OPERATION WARP SPEED

It may seem paradoxical that the Trump administration, stepping back from the federal lead in April 2020, moved that same month to create a powerful federal program to end the pandemic, at least in the United States. The move becomes less mysterious once its origins are better understood.

As NIH scientists rapidly developed a possible design for a COVID-19 vaccine by the middle of January 2020, insiders and outsiders who followed cutting-edge developments in biotechnology sketched ambitious plans. BARDA head Rick Bright, whose job was to develop life-saving drugs and vaccines, had begun brainstorming in the third week of January about crash programs. He had a "horse race" concept of investing in a set of candidates and had already been in touch with leaders of several important companies. That same week, Bright's counterpart working the global side, Richard Hatchett at the Coalition for Epidemic Preparedness Innovation (CEPI), signed a vaccine development contract with Moderna.

We have mentioned that the NSC's Pottinger enlisted Peter Navarro, a Trump adviser on trade and manufacturing, to help him lobby for action. Kicked out of the White House task force after his first appearance there and cued that Bright was working with companies, Navarro reached out to Bright. Early in February, Bright began helping Navarro prepare memos to circulate in the White House and discuss at other NSC meetings.

One of these memos, dated February 9, started off with demands to stop exports of N95 masks and urged the government to lock down supplies of the drug remdesivir. Navarro (and Bright) then proposed "'Manhattan Project' Vaccine Development." The Manhattan Project was the famous army project organized by the U.S. government in 1942 to build the first atomic bomb.[22]

If "we start this week," Navarro (and Bright) argued, workable vaccines might be available by October or November, "with a production capacity of 150 million doses by the end of the year **IF we act NOW**" (emphasis in original). He recommended that the United States invest $1 to 3 billion in a portfolio of four or five candidates, placing contracts within one or two weeks. Bright informed Kadlec that he had helped Navarro develop this idea. The costs being quoted were just for development and trials, not manufacturing or distribution, which would have to be vast enterprises. With Bright's help, Navarro would follow up with other memos on acquisition of needles, syringes, and other vaccine-related supplies.[23]

This proposal stalled, possibly because Kadlec had no money for it until emergency funds started flowing in March, or because it came from Navarro, or because leaders were preoccupied with other matters. One of the participants in the task force remembers that the CDC's Redfield also pushed for such a "Manhattan Project."

In late March, the head regulator of vaccines at FDA, Peter Marks, got involved. He had not participated in any task force meetings. Marks had worked in private industry, understood pharma production, and was troubled about CDC's forecasts of a likely second and more dangerous wave of the virus in the autumn. He thought he saw ways the vaccine development and production process could be greatly accelerated.

Marks reached out to Bright, who shared his planning. With emergency funds flowing, Bright secured money to move forward with a large investment in at least one of the big vaccine candidates, Johnson & Johnson. Kadlec and Azar approved this investment at the end of March, so the issue was on the table.

Meanwhile, also in March, an entrepreneurial outsider, a former secretary of the navy long working on biodefense issues, Richard Danzig, began circulating ideas to accelerate vaccine development. His colleagues in this virtual group included Jeremy Farrar, heading Britain's influential Wellcome Trust foundation; and Paul Stoffels, then a top executive at Johnson & Johnson, and someone who had been working with the government, with Bright.

Also in Danzig's group was Hatchett, another former U.S. official who headed the nonprofit global organization that we have already mentioned, CEPI. Hatchett was trying to develop a slate of possible vaccines for the whole world. With him in this network was a former White House official and private biotech executive, Rajeev Venkayya. Hatchett and Venkayya are members of our group. A public health professor, Marc Lipsitch, and Victor Dzau, the president of the National Academy of Medicine, both members of our group, also joined the discussion.

By late March, Danzig was urging his colleagues to think big about what could be done about the emerging pandemic. After discussions with people in the vaccine industry, Danzig thought that, if paired with "previously unthinkable government support," a vaccine might be prepared in as little as six months, instead of the twelve-to-eighteen-month timeline that others thought was more realistic (which itself would seem ambitious compared to historical practice). He thought such a vaccine should be shared globally and "create immense goodwill and respect for America."[24]

The needed government support, Danzig explained, might include "underwriting costs, indemnification, maximum-speed FDA review, acceptance of additional clinical and manufacturing risk appropriate to the enormous benefit, engagement of reluctant actors, and, if necessary, use of the Defense Production Act."

Farrar recounts this story in his memoir of the crisis. He remembers it as a "Manhattan Project" for vaccines and drugs. Danzig had not used that analogy, but others had. According to Farrar, "Danzig could already see in March 2020 that the obstacles blocking an exit from the pandemic would not be the science but the physical supply of vaccines, from the manufacturing lines down to the availability of glass vials."[25]

Farrar also remembered Danzig's understanding that "if the world wanted vaccines by the end of 2020, it would have to start getting the financing and other pieces of the puzzle, such as manufacturing, scaled up quickly—and all over the world."

To all the members of this group, the costs of action were trivial compared to the costs of inaction—the point economists would later refer to as "spending billions to save trillions." A little later, on May 4, a group of such economists—Susan Athey, Michael Kremer, Christopher Snyder, and Alex Tabarrok—published an opinion piece in the *New York Times* spotlighting an "advance market commitment" strategy. "Today," they wrote, "the U.S. government could go big and create a Covid-19 vaccine [advance market commitment], guaranteeing to spend about $70 billion on new vaccines."[26]

In sum, by early April 2020, the ideas from Bright, Marks, and in Danzig's group had been well circulated and repeatedly discussed among a number of key industry leaders and officials. The circle of officials in Danzig's group included Kadlec in HHS.

On the afternoon of April 10, Marks brainstormed with Kadlec and several of his aides. Marks pitched the idea for a crash government vaccine program. Not only could the government streamline and orchestrate the clinical trials to prove that a vaccine worked, Marks explained, but the government could also do much more to ramp up manufacturing. Marks called for advance market commitments to buy the product. The government could also provide supply chain support to rush vaccines out by the end of the year.

Marks suggested that the whole government could work on this project "in the truest sense of a team." He, like

Danzig, was interested in global sharing. He thought that, working with the nonprofit CEPI headed by Hatchett, such an ambitious project might include the rest of the world. We will return, in chapter 10, to what happened to these plans for a global coalition.[27]

Marks, Kadlec, and Kadlec's staff discussed whether this new program should be called "Manhattan Project 2.0." Marks, a *Star Trek* fan, suggested "Project Warp Speed." That weekend they proposed all of this to Azar.

Azar was sold, completely. The idea came at a time when his own future in the administration hung by a thread. It would bring him and his team into a key role. Azar became a key figure in pushing the project forward. Both Bright and Marks remember working, on Easter weekend, with consultants from the Boston Consulting Group who were helping Azar produce persuasive slide decks that he could use.

Azar persuaded Kushner, helped by one of his aides who was more acceptable to the White House, a former army officer and private healthcare executive and consultant, Paul Mango. Mango became the HHS liaison to the White House.

Kadlec stayed away from the White House, where he knew he was unpopular. Meanwhile, unhappy with Bright for a number of reasons, including arguments about questionable drug approvals and Bright's role in a press leak, Kadlec and Azar pushed Bright out of BARDA and ASPR. Bright soon left the government and filed a whistleblower complaint that was later settled.

In an April 15 meeting with Azar and Mango, Kushner was convinced. He became the liaison to keep President

Trump on board. Trump gave his informal "go ahead" that same day. Operation Warp Speed (which would eventually spend nearly $30 billion) was officially launched on May 15.

We will return to Operation Warp Speed later. What is important to notice now is how remarkably sheltered this program was from the kind of storms that afflicted all other parts of the federal government involved in the crisis. The secretary of defense was Mark Esper. Esper offered his department's help to set up this vaccine program. With help from the Joint Chiefs of Staff chairman, General Mark Milley, they identified their man: a general renowned for his logistic skills, Gustave Perna.

Milley and Perna were old friends. Milley offered his friend the option of retiring from the military and taking the job as a more highly paid civilian contractor. Perna refused, wisely pointing out the value, in getting things done, of a uniformed four-star general visibly taking command. Esper and Milley opened every Pentagon door to what Perna needed, as scores of officers received new orders. Kushner made sure that the same was true at the Office of Management and Budget.

Perna met his partner, who would manage the scientific side of the program, Moncef Slaoui, for the first time at the Rose Garden ceremony where the program was announced. They worked well together from the start. Though they reported regularly on their progress to a board of officials headed by Kushner, both men felt, as they told us very clearly, that they had the autonomy, money, and clarity of purpose they needed in order to do their job. They did not report to the White House task force, which was already dying on the vine.

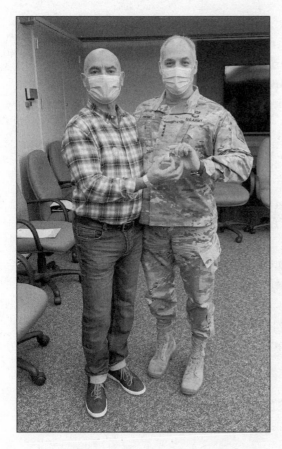

The co-leaders of Operation Warp Speed, Dr. Moncef Slaoui (left) and General Gustave Perna, holding a vial of COVID-19 vaccine prior to receiving their vaccinations.

PHOTO CREDIT: MONCEF SLAOUI

That picture of harmony, authority, and mission stands out in this story like a spotlit actor on a darkened stage. Two possible explanations for this also stand out.

One is that Kushner, through his unusual role in the Trump White House, sheltered the program and its staff from the chaos and cronies. He cut through OMB hesitation to secure the funding—an eye-opening $26 billion request from Perna.

The other, overlapping, explanation is that the Department of Defense and top uniformed officers now played a central role in managing the effort, in Washington and at company offices around the United States. Perna and the defense effort was itself sheltered by General Milley and Secretary Esper.

President Trump would later grouse at all the money going to the companies. But there is no evidence that Kushner had a difficult time; perhaps the promise of a miracle vaccine deflected attention from daily reports of flailing crisis management. Almost everyone would love a miracle vaccine.

But what if the effort failed? Mango has recounted that when Azar first briefed the concept to the White House chief of staff, Meadows, Meadows told Azar: "Alex, if this fails, you will be blamed. If it is successful, you will not get the credit." Azar said he could live with that.[28]

THE BIDEN ADMINISTRATION TAKES OVER

As it took office in January 2021, the Biden administration did not keep the system it inherited. It went back to a system more like the one that the Trump administration had created at the very beginning of March 2020. There was a White House coordinator in a role akin to the one Birx had held, occupied by Jeffrey Zients. Former FDA commissioner David Kessler became the chief science adviser to this task force. That task force then restored a vital federal role in day-to-day crisis management, which had many positive effects.

It helped handle many day-to-day issues. It helped orchestrate deployment of some of the hundreds of billions of dollars that Congress appropriated in the administration's March 2021 American Rescue Plan; money to shore up state and local governments, healthcare providers, public health, and schools.

But the basic trajectory of American government performance in the Covid war was already largely set, as will become clear in the chapters to follow, and the new administration did not fundamentally change it. President Biden seems to have accepted the common belief that the policy problems had stemmed from not "following the science." A group of *Washington Post* reporters interviewed dozens of his officials about how the new president handled the Covid crisis. "He would follow the science, and the science would show the way to ending the pandemic. . . . For months afterward, he had a catchphrase he would use. 'Tell me what to do, docs,' the president would frequently say."[29]

The Biden administration's federal crisis management was more tactical than strategic. It became consumed with managing the battlefields: the situation updates, deployments, and daily problems. The original problem that Anne Schuchat had called strategic-level governance, a function that developed broad policy designs, had still not been solved. The biomedical surveillance challenge had not been addressed.

On testing, Giroir's ad hoc structure had eventually ramped up production of tests. In the second half of 2020, he had focused on buying all the rapid antigen tests that industry could produce, nearly 2 million a day. But that improvised effort lapsed early in the Biden administration.

Production lines wound down; Abbott had to junk millions of tests. Then, during the middle of 2021, the Delta wave, the third wave of the virus, hit. Few tests were available.[30]

"Biden was furious," the *Post* reporters found. "In meetings in the Oval Office, an exasperated Biden repeatedly asked, 'Why didn't we order enough tests? Why didn't we order enough of what we needed?'"

As Omicron, the fourth wave, hit during the winter of 2021–22, the Biden administration organized a massive testing effort, the most comprehensive and well designed effort to date. Early in 2022 they also saw how to link such a program to their strong, if belated, push to find practical ways to reopen schools, a story we describe at the end of our next chapter.

On vaccines, the new team transitioned Operation Warp Speed back to HHS at the beginning of 2022 in a new organization, meant to be much more operational and initially led by a veteran operator, Jason Roos. The organization is called H-CORE, for HHS Coordination Operations and Response Element. It was meant to supplement BARDA and help acquire and distribute tests, drugs, and vaccines.

H-CORE is an important experiment to test whether HHS can import the management and operational skills it relied on, during the Covid war, from FEMA and then from the Department of Defense. Its "peacetime" future is still unclear. The ASPR has also been elevated, during 2022, into an operational division on par with the CDC, FDA, and NIH. But that change does little to clarify what role it may play in the next crisis, in relation to the other power centers in HHS and the rest of the government.

6

COMMUNITIES IMPROVISE WITH FEW TOOLS

IN THE UNITED STATES OF AMERICA, federal crisis leadership receded or vanished during the spring of 2020. One quite capable local public health leader described this to us as feeling like she was "watching a giant boulder rolling downhill" right at her and her community.

As April 2020 began, the "15 Days to Slow the Spread" came to an end. But the spread did not slow down, and every community in America prepared to defend itself.

State and local authorities felt they were on their own. This wasn't their imagination. As we mentioned, on March 21, Jared Kushner, President Trump's son-in-law and senior adviser, had told a gathering of private sector officials: "The federal government is not going to lead this response. It's up to the states to figure out what they want to do." At the same time, President Trump was privately telling Bob Woodward: "You know, it's a local problem. You can't solve that federally."[1] One of our members, a former public health official out in the field, said it reminded her of *The Hunger Games*. "It was like there was an invasion on U.S. soil by a foreign adversary and the White House was telling all fifty governors, 'Good luck. You're on your own, and now you're also fighting each other for weapons and supplies.'"

Usually led by governors and mayors, leaders improvised new, ad hoc setups to manage their Covid wars. The communities faced a cascade of terribly difficult choices. The ones that did best

- figured out how to work together in fusion cells, sharing daily information and organizing actions across agencies;
- used blunt instruments when community spread was at its worst, while they
- devised better, more surgical, toolkits to make people feel safer returning to school or work.

As their state's public health institutions were quickly overwhelmed, the common response of these governors and other leaders, played out in dozens of ways, was to create ad hoc governance. They enlisted businesspeople they or their friends knew. They reached out to leaders at their major metro medical centers. They recruited contractors and consultants to do a lot of the work.

Take, for example, the state of Connecticut. Governor Ned Lamont created the Reopen Connecticut committee. It was co-chaired by a former top PepsiCo executive, Indra Nooyi, and a senior epidemiologist at Yale, Albert Ko. We talked to them both. They began frantically identifying and enlisting stakeholders, including in the business community, and developing plans for what to do and how to communicate about it. We heard similar stories from people in many other states around the country.

A standard style of research in public health and medicine relies on hindsight to compare outcomes, to determine what worked and what didn't. People don't make policy this way, of course. Even if they did, prescriptions from some past crisis may not be readily applicable to a new context.

FROM FLYING BLIND TO FUSION CELLS

As we tried to reconstruct how these choices were made at the time, the first point to stress is how little information these people had about the danger. In the spring of 2020, they were flying blind. They had little reliable information about where and how quickly the virus was spreading. When they saw the chaos unfolding in Italian and New York City hospitals, they feared the pandemic might overwhelm their entire healthcare system. Their natural and understandable tendency was to urge people to, in effect, shelter in place, if they could.

On March 19, the governor of California became the first governor to close all nonessential businesses and order residents to remain at home. Around the same time, the governor of Ohio closed all K-12 public schools for in-person learning. Within two weeks, every governor except one (South Dakota) had issued similar orders.

The United States was not alone. Beginning in mid-March 2020, lockdowns and broad closures were common around the world. Much of the entire United States remained under stay-at-home orders throughout most of the month of April.

Officials told us that, at the time, they thought these extreme emergency measures would probably be in place only for a few weeks. They thought these temporary decrees would be lifted once everyone had a better grasp of what to do or the height of the emergency had passed. In the Crimson Contagion exercise that we mentioned at the beginning of the previous chapter, the assumption was that, as people came out of their shelters, a plan would be ready for treatment, healthcare, and emergency management.

Weeks passed, but the pandemic only grew worse. Nonetheless, in May 2020 some top officials, including in the White House, started believing that the worst had passed. There were lively disagreements among experts about what to expect in the fall of 2020 and winter of 2020–21. Some of the more worried experts, including some of the Wolverines, believed the worst was still to come. They turned out to be right. The main killing season for the virus in the United States came in the later waves.

During those waves, officials realized that tools like contact tracing and monitored quarantines could not work well for mitigation and suppression. The substantial asymptomatic and pre-symptomatic spread of the virus meant that contact tracing approaches that worked for some other diseases were less effective. Where community spread was unstoppable, contact tracing was not the best use of scarce people. Writing to Anthony Fauci in January 2021, Marcelle Layton, head of the bureau of communicable disease at New York City's health department, noted that "few of our

[COVID] cases occur among persons who were already known contacts under monitoring."[2]

The best that authorities could do was pool their resources and do the best biomedical surveillance in their communities that they could, updated daily. Then, still working together, they could give the community continuing guidance that tailored actions to the changing situation.

Once again consider, for example, the German story. The German success with containment during the spring of 2020 did not shield it from a devastating spread of the virus during the fall and winter of 2020–21. During that period, their contact tracing was also often overwhelmed.

What the Germans had, though, was superior testing and biomedical surveillance, which gave the authorities and public more confidence that they knew what was going on. Policymakers felt more in control, with less of a sense that they were constantly on the back foot. That carried into their public communication. This, in turn, enhanced public support and compliance, even though many Germans were also resentful of lockdowns and argued about the diverging approaches adopted by their different states.[3]

Given this greater situation awareness, throughout the crisis the German states had fewer school closures than in the United States and their business lockdowns were more targeted. When the second wave hit, in fall 2020, German caregivers had had time to absorb lessons in best clinical practices, making the standard of care stronger. During the first phase, the Germans had done a good job of protecting nursing homes and other especially vulnerable sites, which helped them better cope when these defenses were more challenged.

If American officials at least had a good crisis management process, pooling and sharing information in a clear way, people in the community would have been able to understand their dilemmas a little better, empathizing with their difficult choices and feeling that their leaders were on top of the situation.

One of our listening sessions was with nine people from the McChrystal Group, including its head, retired general Stan McChrystal. As crisis management consultants, they had helped organize improvised processes in Boston, in Missouri, in Virginia, and in Nebraska, and participated in the State and Territory Alliance for Testing group organized by the Rockefeller Foundation. They helped stand up "fusion cells," organizing hundreds of people who met almost every day, week in week out, month in month out. The cells spotlighted problems. They emphasized transparency about what had been decided and what was going to happen. They pointed up accountability among the people who were to make things happen.

In a typical state, it was not unusual for more than a dozen different state agencies to be engaged. Sharing their experiences, the McChrystal Group's principals had found that, often, there was confusion about who had authority. Social media contributed to that confusion.

Part of the job was just to develop a common picture of what was going on, and update that picture every day. The data systems were "pathetic." Then came the tasks. "People were trying to do the right thing," one member of the group also told us, "but they didn't know how." Speed was essential. Some private firms just started donating technology to help. Different parts of a state had different problems. So, usually, the work had to zero in on local health districts. Often it was the state's emergency management agency that had more experience in acting during a crisis, if they could team up with other relevant institutions, public and private.

The Covid war forced emergency managers to create the kinds of fusion cells that agencies ordinarily resisted in peacetime. A similar experience occurred for terrorism emergencies after the 9/11 shock of 2001. At the local level, more attention was given to regular operation of first responder incident command systems and to Joint Terrorism Task Forces. Those joint efforts rolled up to the newly created National Counterterrorism Center at the federal level that, over the last twenty years, has been widely regarded as one of the more successful innovations to emerge from that crisis.

LOCKDOWNS AND "METRICS" IN THE SPRING AND SUMMER OF 2020: "RED" AND "BLUE" FACE COMMON DILEMMAS

The whole nation locked down during the second half of March 2020. The problem was what to do next, in April, May, and beyond.

Shutdowns can slow the spread of a pandemic, but they also damage the economy, undermine education, worsen psychological problems, and defer needed maintenance of all kinds, including medical treatment. In short, they inflict a high price.

By May, governors throughout the country recognized that lockdowns were no longer sustainable. They needed to try something else. At the time, they perceived a trade-off:

either they could protect public health or they could protect their local economies. In practice, they had to do both, but the balance was hard to strike.

As we observed earlier, in April 2020 President Trump and some of his advisers began convincing themselves that the pandemic was subsiding and would not be such a big deal. The public health leaders, like Birx and the CDC experts, were not so optimistic.

The rosy scenario started fading with the end of springtime. In the summer of 2020, the first wave of infections spread further around the country. Many health experts were even more worried—correctly—about what the fall and winter would bring.

But, after the March lockdown, those experts did not have very good ideas about what to do next.

President Trump was encouraging America to reopen. He then stepped back from the painful trade-offs of how to do that. His administration, divided and snarled, became more detached from the real decisions about whether or how to reopen.

Meanwhile, without a system of biomedical surveillance, policymakers were still flying blind until people started showing up in emergency rooms. The health experts were still arguing about asymptomatic spread and how the virus was transmitted. It was not clear how much lockdowns would slow community spread. State and local leaders were anxious, correctly as we will show in the next chapter, about whether their fraying healthcare systems could stand any large margin of added strain.

In the first months of the pandemic, there was no option of just reopening and accepting the risk. Even if governments did nothing, anxious people would change their behavior. Nor was there an option of just isolating everyone indefinitely. The economic, educational, and psychological costs of isolation were not easily weighed against physical health risks, but all were real.

The wisest policymakers had to face up to the dilemma. There were no ideal answers. Competence meant acknowledging the necessary balancing acts, with all their imperfections, and then devising practical approaches in between the poles of shutting society down or pretending there was no problem.

The Germans' success in 2020 was not that they found the perfect policy formula. It was that their government tended to work the problem in a more organized, practical, and proactive way. They made rapid decisions about how to strike a balance, gave out protocols to implement those decisions, balanced the risks, and monitored what happened.

One interesting finding from the data about comparative American and European performance is that, during the first wave of the virus in the spring and summer of 2020, European excess mortality was 29 percent lower than that in the United States. In other words, they did better, but not enormously better. The difference may partly be explained by the differences in quality of containment policies (chapter 4), including biomedical surveillance and use of testing, and overall crisis management (chapter 5). The differences in performance would get much larger as the pandemic went on, and the likely mix of reasons for these differences would shift.[4]

In the first wave, in the spring and summer of 2020, many American authorities learned the lessons about how to accept and balance risks, but they had to learn them the hard way. They all tended to come around to the view that they needed to lift or impose restrictions based on "metrics" of sickness in their communities.

Based on the false notion of a trade-off, which became common during April and May 2020, governors made their choices. Some governors (mostly Republicans) chose to prioritize their local economies, while others (mostly Democrats) chose to prioritize public health.

Anyone listening to the noisy debate that followed might have concluded that in May 2020 Republican governors suddenly flipped a switch, ended their lockdowns, and reopened their economies, while Democratic governors kept their states in the total darkness of lockdowns for many more months. *That is not what really happened.*

While Republicans and Democrats differed somewhat in their approaches, the entire country began to emerge from lockdown in May 2020. Most Democratic governors began relaxing restrictions around the same time that Republican governors began to do so.

Democratic governors were more cautious than their Republican counterparts. They tended to relax restrictions more gradually. They did not commit to dates for reopening. They preferred, instead, to wait and see how the pandemic evolved.

Like Democrats, most Republican governors began to lift restrictions gradually, in phases, but their timetables were aggressive. Most planned to fully reopen within a few weeks, by the end of May or early June. Many Republican governors quickly discovered these timetables were unrealistic. Some states reopened on schedule in May and remained open for the duration of the pandemic, but many others did not. Texas was typical. By early June 2020, Texas had entered phase 3 of a four-phase reopening plan, which meant that all businesses in the state were open, with some occupancy limitations. Within a few weeks, as summer arrived and before the state could move to phase 4, the virus surged. It forced Texas to pause its reopening, close some businesses, and impose new restrictions.

When the surge subsided in the fall, Texas resumed efforts to reopen. It had to pause again in December when the virus surged for its second and especially deadly wave. The governor did not proclaim that Texas was "100 percent open" until March 2021.

This Texas story was not unusual. Many states that began to reopen in May 2020 were forced later to pause or even retreat and were unable to complete the reopening process until late 2020 or early 2021. By that time, most Democratic governors had reopened their businesses too.

In 2020, successive waves of pandemic forced most governors, Republican and Democrat, to endure what one author has described as "the hammer and the dance." During the first wave, governors used the "hammer," or lockdowns. But, as that wave rippled across the country during the summer, lockdowns were no longer an option. Instead, governors had to learn to "dance" with the virus. When the virus surged, they imposed restrictions. As it receded, they relaxed restrictions. When it surged again, they reimposed the restrictions.[5]

A common fallacy among critics of lockdowns is to assume that, if the rules on reopening changed, everything would go back to normal. The people were not sheep. Studies indicate that, regardless of how the rules were changing, a lot of citizens were doing their own version of the hammer and the dance. When the virus worsened, people were more fearful and were more careful. When the virus seemed to ease, they eased up, too.[6]

All governors, Republican and Democrat, used the toolkit of restrictions. In the absence of federal leadership, in December 2020 governors from both parties, representing one-third of Americans, even joined a common "Call to Action," working with the nonprofit Covid Collaborative, to agree on a common approach. Most governors closed high-contact businesses, like bars, restaurants, and gyms. They imposed occupancy limitations on businesses. They limited large gatherings and required travelers arriving from high-risk states to quarantine.[7]

One of us, Alex Lazar, was involved in many of the state improvisations. He remembers the experience very well. "I attended a ton (I still attend—now up to maybe 250+ of these) of multi-state (up to thirty-five states represented—blue, red, and whatever is in between) planning/sharing meetings where we discussed very frankly Covid management and communication issues."

"Our conversations," Lazar recalled, "were stripped of politics as these were operational meetings. Thus, politics were addressed as operational constraints rather than moral imperatives. What impressed me most about these very frank discussions is that almost everyone was well within a standard deviation of what everyone else was doing. It was more of a purple bell curve than a bimodal distribution of red and blue peaks."

Yes, there were differences in public presentation. But "it was how these policies were communicated that differed

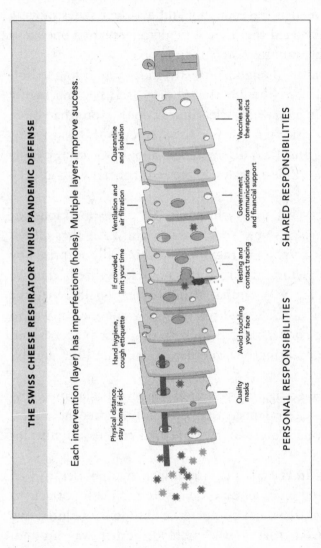

THE SWISS CHEESE RESPIRATORY VIRUS PANDEMIC DEFENSE

Each intervention (layer) has imperfections (holes). Multiple layers improve success.

Physical distance, stay home if sick

Quality masks

Hand hygiene, cough etiquette

Avoid touching your face

If crowded, limit your time

Testing and contact tracing

Ventilation and air filtration

Government communications and financial support

Quarantine and isolation

Vaccines and therapeutics

PERSONAL RESPONSIBILITIES

SHARED RESPONSIBILITIES

A diagram of the "Swiss cheese" model of pandemic defense. Each intervention, such as masking or distancing or vaccines, can be thought of as a piece of Swiss cheese, with various holes. Layering multiple interventions helps to fill the holes and improve success.

ADAPTED FROM IAN M. MACKAY AT WWW.VIROLOGYDOWNUNDER.COM

more than the substance of what happened. Red [officials] stated that they were doing a phased operation because we wanted to reopen the economy and get their states moving again. Blues stated that they were doing a phased operation because they want to protect their people."

In substance, though, "honestly, most were trying to 'follow the science' (though this phrase itself became highly politicized in a very non-scientific fashion)—some had more appetite for risk than others. However, even this was not as stark as it seems. Reds always talked about protecting people as well and Blues always expressed concerns about the economy."

"As I traveled to Washington, DC, Austin, Houston, Boston, Chicago, New York, Tampa, and LA—they all felt very similar despite the rhetoric. I was initially surprised by this as the rhetoric was so different." He realized "that we were all doing very similar things operationally." A great untold story of the Covid war was how common it was to find selfless cooperation, people sharing best practices and regularly supporting one another across state lines and all political persuasions.

Further investigation will probably reveal that some governors were better dancers than others. But, after the successive pandemic waves, every state had suffered significant casualties.

To be clear: there is a common view that politics, a "Red response" and a "Blue response," were the main obstacle to protecting citizens, not competence and policy failures. We found, instead, that it was more the other way around. Incompetence and policy failures, including the failure of federal executive leadership, produced bad outcomes, flying blind, and resorting to blunt instruments. Those failures and tensions fed toxic politics that further divided the country in a crisis rather than bringing it together.

These divisions then played out in the world of scholars. In October 2020, debates featured competing declarations: the Great Barrington Declaration and the John Snow Memorandum, each signed by thousands of supporters.

"Great Barrington" supporters called for "focused protection" of the vulnerable and a return to normal life for everyone else, which would accelerate evolution of "herd immunity" across the whole population. "John Snow" signers did not think it was feasible to identify and segregate the vulnerable; nor did they have as much faith in herd immunity. For them, the best approach was to protect all of society through continued "evidence-based" mitigation measures.

These dueling abstractions of October 2020 were another symptom of policy failure. In practice, governors needed a better toolkit. They needed one with more precision tools that would allow them to dissect risk and avoid blanket shutdowns.

THE ALTERNATIVE—MORE SURGICAL TOOLKITS TO HELP AND REASSURE PEOPLE

Many Americans began forming a bad image of public health—that it was about negative regulation, closing things down. *The whole point of the toolkits, however, should have been to present public health as a positive aid to reopen America.*

The toolkits could help people feel it was reasonably safe to go back to school and go to work. The toolkits might or

POTENTIAL POLICY TOOLS	POTENTIAL FOCAL POINTS
Masking	Healthcare Facilities
Social Distancing	Nursing Homes
Remote School/Work	Schools and Universities
Isolation/Quarantine	Childcare Facilities
Lockdowns	Communities at Risk
Surveillance Testing	Workplaces
Diagnostic Testing	Transportation
Contact Tracing	Restaurants and Bars
Travel Bans	Retail Outlets
Wastewater Surveillance	Places of Worship
Air Ventilation	Entertainment Venues
Paid Sick Leave	
Financial Assistance	

A chart showing non-pharmaceutical policy tools and where they might be deployed. This is an example of the toolkit available to policymakers before vaccines and therapeutics are widely available in an infectious disease crisis. Policymakers can mix and match policy tools and apply them to where they will be most effective.

might not actually help curb community spread. They could, though, show that schools and workplaces were just as safe, if not safer, than anyplace else they could go. This is a fundamental insight for any strategy that relies on extended use of these non-medical tools.

One of us, James Lawler, an experienced infectious disease expert, told us that "Lockdowns are blunt sledgehammers and should NEVER be used unless in the most desperate of circumstances. We can implement targeted and limited interventions that reduce indoor exposure, large gatherings, enforce (and provide) face masks and hygiene—we will get to >90% of the impact for <10% of the collateral damage."

Another one of us, Danielle Allen at Harvard, working with a colleague at Microsoft, Glen Weyl, organized a group to work on toolkits. They got started in March 2020. They saw that the American debate seemed to pose a false choice between public health and economic health. "In fact, lockdowns were not an active policy themselves but mostly an unavoidable and largely organic response to *failed* policy."

Allen started with a core group of nine people, networking with other colleagues, meeting almost every day throughout that spring. They started adding a mayors' group, working with the Rockefeller Foundation. They had a legislative group, working with Congress. She and Weyl later explained: "In the U.S. in March and April public debate focused on a choice between lockdowns to preserve public health and opening to revive the economy. This was a fruitless debate. The international experience largely belied any such trade-off. . . . The countries that performed best on public health also suffered the least economic damage."

It will take time to sift the lessons from all the state and local choices. All we can offer at this point are our impressions, based on some data but not enough.

We think some communities did better than others. For instance, all of New England—Massachusetts, the city of Boston, Connecticut, Rhode Island, New Hampshire, Vermont, and Maine—seem to us to have done relatively well, including their ad hoc crisis management setups. Maine, for instance, had the oldest median age in the country, but was one of the best states in performance. The New England leaders included both Republicans and Democrats.

The state of Washington seems to have done well, partly aided by exceptionally strong public-private partnerships coordinated by an organization called Challenge Seattle. The leader of Challenge Seattle, former Washington governor Christine Gregoire, told us that "[t]he private sector saved the day. Amazon, Microsoft, Boeing, Starbucks, and other Washington-based companies were all very helpful." Not only did these companies share substantial supply-chain know-how with the public sector, but "[s]tate officials learned from the experiences of these companies in other countries" due to their presence overseas. This is a pattern we also saw repeated in much of Canada. Moreover, when these Seattle companies saw what was happening in China and shut down very early, Gregoire believes that they "sent a message to the rest of the community."

The city of Houston also appeared to do relatively well when compared to other similarly sized metropolitan areas. In Houston, as in some parts of Florida, prior experience with emergency management in hurricanes and floods seemed to have a big positive impact on interagency cooperation in this emergency too. Some states, like California, were so large and diverse, and had such a relatively weak state-level public health system, that their performance varied quite a lot from county to county.

One feature we noticed about states that did relatively well is that they immediately developed toolkits and, in late

2020 and early 2021, as more tools became available, they made them even more surgical. For example, by the spring of 2020 experts realized that nursing homes were one of their most important concerns. So, as more tests became available, some health leaders encouraged "point of care" testing to at least provide extra screening and protection to those sites.

Most toolkits have some common features:

- Provide transparent communication about the risks and ways to stay safer, including use of quality masks, made available en masse.

- Regulate mass gatherings, especially indoors.

- Create guidelines and resources to make workplaces and schools safer, mainly with screening (once rapid antigen tests became available), ventilation, use of smaller work or student "cohorts," and masking.

- Set up screening stations both for the community *and* to screen people in workplaces and schools, to allow those testing negative to participate and get retested when appropriate, what some called "test to stay."

- Protect concentrations of the most vulnerable people, above all in nursing facilities, hospitals and clinics, and prisons.

This last point deserves extra emphasis.

Historically, the health burden of an epidemic or pandemic falls unevenly across the population. Some groups were more susceptible to Covid because they were elderly or had comorbidities like heart disease, lung disease, diabetes, and obesity. Some groups had a higher risk of exposure to disease because they lived in densely populated urban areas, multi-family housing, or overcrowded households. Some groups were more likely to use public transportation or work in public-facing jobs, like transportation, healthcare, and food services. Some groups didn't have timely access to high-quality healthcare. They lacked health insurance or a regular source of healthcare. They didn't speak English or may have been deterred from seeking care because of past discrimination or fear of deportation.

While many groups were unusually vulnerable to the COVID-19 pandemic, three stand out.

With an average age in the eighties, nursing home residents were exceptionally vulnerable to poor outcomes from Covid. Many had multiple comorbidities or compromised immune systems, predisposing them to even higher rates of hospitalization and death.

In addition, the close-quarters living situation of nursing home residents made them more likely to get infected than elderly citizens living independently. They shared living, sleeping, and bathing spaces, and many received one-on-one care, such as assistance with bathing or dressing, which did not allow for social distancing. Staff and caregivers, some of whom worked in multiple nursing homes, frequently came in and out of the building, bringing the virus with them. Dwindling Medicaid reimbursement rates and poor oversight from state regulatory agencies meant that these facilities were unprepared to protect their residents from this new threat.

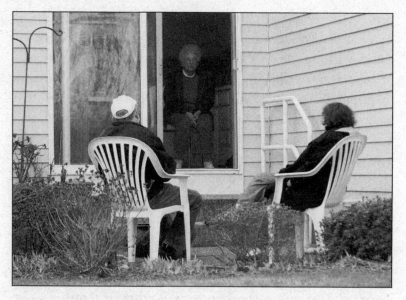

A son-in-law and daughter visit her mother while practicing social distancing at a senior housing development on April 5, 2020, in East Meadow, New York. This scene played out in communities across the United States during the first year of the pandemic.
PHOTO CREDIT: BRUCE BENNET/GETTY IMAGES

Many states sought to protect nursing home residents by, for example, closing facilities to visitors. Cut off from close contact with family and friends, these residents undoubtedly suffered and, despite these restrictions, in the first year of the pandemic more than one out of ten nursing home residents died from COVID-19. Estimates vary, but during the first wave of the virus as many as 20 to 50 percent of the Covid deaths may have come from nursing homes.[8]

Essential workers, outside of the healthcare system, were also at high risk of infection from COVID-19 but received very little protection. Early in the pandemic, states designated many workers as "essential" and ordered them to continue working. At that time there were no federal standards or regulations requiring employers to protect these workers from exposure to COVID-19, nor were there tools to help well-meaning businesses of all sizes meet such standards. Essential workers often worked in crowded conditions without adequate personal protective equipment.

Many worked in low-wage or temporary jobs where they were not entitled to paid sick leave, which presented daily dilemmas for American workers and their families. If they worked while sick with Covid, that increased the risks that the virus would spread in their workplaces. If they contracted the virus but stayed home, they might be fired. And if they quit their job to protect themselves and their families, they might not be entitled to unemployment compensation. Even workers with paid sick leave would quickly exhaust whatever leave they had, making them vulnerable for the remainder of the year (including when childcare became unreliable and even unavailable due to Covid). The lack of routine testing and screening made it difficult or impossible for businesses to distinguish Covid from other illnesses, and prevent the spread of Covid at their places of work.

Before COVID-19, history demonstrated that a third set of groups—African Americans, Hispanics, and American Indians—was vulnerable in a public health emergency. Historically, these groups had long had less access to healthcare, thus less access to testing, vaccination, and treatment. During the H1N1 epidemic in 2009, African Americans and Hispanics had disproportionately higher rates of infection and complications than other groups. African Americans had more comorbidities that made them susceptible to infections. Even controlling for this factor, their outcomes were far worse than for the population as a whole. Spanish-speaking Hispanics had greater exposure risks and less access to healthcare. COVID-19 exposed African Americans and Hispanics to even greater risks, because so many of them were essential workers.[9]

SHIFTING FROM "SLOW THE SPREAD" TO "HOW TO REOPEN"

During the late spring and summer of 2020, most guidelines for reopening were metrics about community spread. But, by the autumn of 2020, this was changing. Several nonpolitical private groups and foundations, including Danielle Allen's team, emphasized that "slow the spread" had become the wrong mantra for community defense. The principal objective should have been to help people get back to work and go to school *even if community spread remained high*.

With this objective, the strategy could shift. The metrics or stoplight charts of community spread would become less important.

The main tools would be screening tests, improved air circulation, and masks. We have compared, for example, the schools guidelines issued by Allen and her partners in July 2020, December 2020, and March 2021 with the CDC guidelines issued throughout this period. The side-by-side comparisons are striking.[10]

The CDC guidelines shifted very slowly and presented practical problems to those trying to interpret them. They did not strongly emphasize either practical ideas for screening testing or improved air quality until well into 2021.

We have heard conflicting assertions about America's capacity to provide adequate PCR testing during the late spring and summer of 2020. Everyone agrees that the PCR tests were the gold standard for spotting a current or recent infection. They were expensive. It took time to process them, often more than seventy-two hours. As more tests were manufactured during the summer of 2020, the turnaround times to process results got longer. The lab capacity could not keep up with the volume.

Simpler, much cheaper, and much faster rapid antigen testing started to show great promise. There are good questions, which we cannot resolve, about whether the U.S. government did all it could to develop these tests, clear them through the FDA approval process, and make them available.

The antigen tests cost about one-tenth as much as the PCR tests and could provide results in about fifteen minutes. They rarely had any false positives. They did have some false negatives—they missed some people who were infected, especially those who were early in the infection or were asymptomatic cases. But, although the PCR test was best for clinical diagnosis, the antigen test had value for screening. It detected a degree of infectiousness that meant that person was capable of spreading the virus.

Worldwide, good rapid antigen tests were being developed by big companies like Abbott, Roche, Thermo Fisher,

Siemens, and Becton Dickinson, and smaller labs were developing other innovative ways to carry out these tests. But these rapid antigen tests did not become available until the summer of 2020, and they were not available on a large scale until the fall of 2020. The U.S. government committed to buy all the antigen tests that Abbott could produce, 150 million of them, between August and December 2020.[11]

Once rapid antigen testing became available on a large scale, during the fall of 2020, it was easier to develop targeted screening to protect workplaces and schools. Even if tests were mass produced, leaders had to design and implement operational concepts for how to use these tools practically, at scale, in the field, for broad biomedical surveillance and protection of workplaces or schools. In the United States, this potential was not properly exploited. Why?

We are not confident we know the answers. The question may need more investigation than we could conduct. The relevant federal leadership—Birx and Giroir as well as Redfield and CDC leaders—all seem to have supported massive use of antigen tests. It was true that antigen tests were not as sensitive as PCR tests. But in a crisis, and especially for screening, fast and available was better than slow (PCR) or nothing.

Leaders debated strategies for deploying tens of millions of tests—mass population biomedical surveillance, point of care in vulnerable population groups, and screening at schools or workplaces. Even in the fall of 2020 there were not enough antigen tests to do all these things. Given the circumstances, we think the last two strategies should have had the highest priority. In practice, most decisions about what to do were left with the states once they got their allocation of available tests.

In addition to the numbers problem, the antigen tests faced a problem of state acceptance. Giroir told investigators that the problem with antigen testing was mostly with what he called "lab snobs" who "really believed that the only appropriate test was a molecular PCR test done by a naso-pharyngeal swab that was sent to a central laboratory because that was—it wasn't the gold standard; it was a standard." But they thought the "'gold standard' for an individual diag-nosis was the only thing [that] could be used from a public health point of view." Some of us experienced what Giroir described.[12]

Yet another problem was at the federal level, centered at the FDA. The FDA's center that handled testing did slowly approve guidelines that would allow enterprising doctors to order antigen tests for screening purposes. But the FDA did not provide plain, broad approval for the use of such tests in asymptomatic cases *until the spring of 2021*. Without such clarity, many state and local health authorities were reluctant to authorize such screening tests; some insurers were reluc-tant to pay for them.[13]

In sum, what was missing was a strong, clear, written articulation of a national strategy for how to use antigen or PCR tests for workplaces and schools. Such a strategy would explain what the antigen tests in these plans were expected to do. That could then be lined up, in writing, with the FDA's regulatory position. These plans would then be com-bined with an understanding of how this approach could be financed by the end-users, and it should have been ready by the fall of 2020. The Biden administration finally designed such a comprehensive program, which it deployed in the first months of 2022.

We were impressed by the Rapid Screening Consortium developed in Canada by a research group at the University of Toronto called the Creative Destruction Lab. Set up in August 2020, with support from some of Canada's leading companies, its goal was to bring build a robust rapid screening system that could be implemented at scale so that Canada's economy could reopen and stay open.

A dozen companies kicked in enough money to launch the project with a budget of several million dollars. The consortium, which included Canada's leading airline, Air Canada, pooled people and resources to get tests, build a data system (in partnership with Microsoft) to report the anonymized results of rapid tests, and use the updates to drive policy. Pilot sites launched in January 2021. During that year, as Canada's government public health system tottered and stopped PCR testing, the consortium kept growing and growing. Eventually thousands of companies were participating.

By using rapid antigen tests for screening, the burden on PCR testing was eased. If a positive antigen test result was confirmed, people followed public health guidance to stay home for five days or until they were asymptomatic, in which case they could test again and, if negative, go back to work. In this Canadian program, people with positive diagnoses received sick leave. Paid sick leave was not so available in American toolkits, especially among the most vulnerable essential workers.

IMPROVING AIR QUALITY:
THE MISJUDGMENT ON AEROSOL SPREAD

In any war, one of the most important jobs is to assess the nature of the enemy. In the Covid war, that meant assessing the virus, how it spread, whether and where it had spread in the United States, and how it was evolving.

The first critical period to do this assessment was in the couple of months between mid-January and mid-March 2020. As we mentioned earlier, the United States could not get critical information out of China.

The most important and fundamental misjudgment about the viral enemy was about how it spread. Early on, the U.S. government and the WHO mistakenly assessed that the virus was transmitted on surfaces, or large respiratory droplets, and that aerosol transmission was rare. The truth was just the opposite.[14]

Experts, including the Wolverines network, were already calling out this misjudgment and pressing the case for aerosol transmission. Two of us, Michael Callahan and James Lawler, were treating patients on the stricken *Diamond Princess* cruise ship in February 2020 and noticed evidence of aerosol transmission. Lawler saw the same thing in his medical center. Another one of us, Mike Osterholm, was also arguing that aerosol transmission was the key. A number of other experts were pressing their case by March 2020, partly from analysis of some of the cruise ship evidence, their own observations, and evidence from outbreaks in meatpacking and processing plants. Then came a remarkable outbreak in May 2020 from a choir practice in Washington State.[15]

Yet the opposing view dominated CDC and WHO guidance through most of 2020. At least until April 2020, and intermittently after that, this mistaken assessment also downplayed the significance of air quality and ventilation. As most Americans remember, what ensued instead was a frenzy of deep cleaning in every part of America. This "hygiene theater" likely contributed little if anything to reducing the spread of the virus.

It is hard to overstate the significance of this misjudgment in framing policy tools and undermining public confidence in expert guidance throughout the rest of 2020 and into 2021, the deadliest and most costly phase of the pandemic in the United States. Sociologist Zeynep Tufekci put it well when she discussed the issue in May 2021:

> If the importance of aerosol transmission had been accepted early, we would have been told from the beginning that it was much safer outdoors, where these small particles disperse more easily, as long as you avoid close, prolonged contact with others. We would have tried to make sure indoor spaces were well ventilated, with air filtered as necessary. Instead of blanket rules on gatherings, we would have targeted conditions that can produce superspreading events: people in poorly ventilated indoor spaces, especially if engaged over time in activities that would increase aerosol production, like shouting and singing. We would have started using masks more quickly, and we would have paid more attention to their fit, too. And we would have been less obsessed with cleaning surfaces. Our mitigations would have been

much more effective, sparing us a great deal of suffering and anxiety.[16]

This misjudgment was disproportionately American. Public health authorities from other nations picked up the clues on the aerosol threat much more quickly. They then implemented policies that dramatically curtailed community transmission.

A notable example was Japan. There public health authorities launched their "Three C's" campaign of awareness in early March 2020. The Three C's campaign instructed citizens to avoid (1) crowded places, (2) closed spaces, and (3) close-contact settings. That was based on the assessment of Japanese public health experts that the virus might be transmitted by surface or airborne routes, often by asymptomatic individuals, and that epidemic growth was driven by sporadic superspreading events, facilitated by large indoor gatherings. While definitive and scientifically indisputable evidence was still lacking, Japanese public health officials were willing to make these proclamations based upon the preponderance of evidence and their professional judgment.[17]

The result in Japan was a campaign that likely saved many tens of thousands of lives, compared to the anemic guidance coming out of the United States. They also accomplished this without U.S.-level lockdowns or severe restrictions in citizen movement and in-person schooling. Despite 2022's increases in Covid deaths in Japan due to relaxed mitigation measures and Omicron-related variants, Japan's cumulative Covid mortality per capita remains almost a *tenth* that of the United States.

But it is not enough to just call out the aerosol misjudgment. We and others have tried to understand it.

Groups of scholars led by Katherine Randall and Jose-Luis Jimenez explain this misjudgment by digging into the insular history and methods of the expert community that has studied infectious respiratory disease for more than a hundred years, who had come to accept a too-neat separation of "droplets" and "aerosols." They had adopted an arbitrary threshold for separating these categories, mainly from work past scientists had done on tuberculosis. The work of other scientists, used to working on occupational safety issues or in fields of biology and agricultural science where aerosol issues are old hat, did not make much of a dent in the received wisdom.[18]

After the U.S. invasion of Iraq in 2003, when it became clear that many U.S. and allied intelligence assessments of Iraq's weapons of mass destruction had turned out to be catastrophically wrong, the CIA conducted its own searching and critical evaluation of its methods. A presidential commission did the same. So did a Senate committee.

We are not suggesting that these failures of intelligence assessment are equivalent. But both episodes illustrate the risks that go with reliance on vital intelligence assessments by an insular intellectual community that does not reflect enough on its own analytical tradecraft and does not deliberately foster alternative views.

These failures also reflected poorly on the organizational culture of public health agencies in the United States, particularly at the CDC. Some individual experts at CDC had strong suspicions that airborne spread might also be crucial, as well as the scale of asymptomatic transmission and other key features the Japanese had acted upon so promptly. Indeed, the CDC had some of the most technically gifted experts in the world. Yet the culture of the organization, emphasizing certainty before action, resulted in paralysis.

These misjudgments about aerosols slowed use of one crucial tool—emphasizing the relative safety of outdoor activities and the role of air changes and ventilation, and even led to the sometimes ludicrous warnings about outdoor activity. They also fed uncertainty about the significance of masks. But even where good masks were available, many governors were reluctant, largely for political reasons, to use that tool.

THE PROBLEMS WITH MASKS

As soon as the danger from airborne transmission became evident, masks were an obvious precaution. Scientific studies steadily validated this precaution, while emphasizing the value of high-quality masks.[19]

Because of the misjudgments about aerosol spread and fears about shortages of masks, leading public health voices cautioned against their use in the formative early weeks of the pandemic. The surgeon general, Jerome Adams, sent out a widely noted tweet in February: "Seriously people— STOP BUYING MASKS! They are NOT effective in preventing general public from catching #Coronavirus, but if healthcare providers can't get them to care for sick patients, it puts them and our communities at risk." During that phase, Fauci and Birx were not mask advocates. The CDC did not recommend their use among asymptomatic people until April.[20]

In the first months of the crisis, good masks were scarce. Much of the world had outsourced production of many medical supplies and pharmaceuticals to China. Had China not contained its Covid pandemic early on, the supply crisis would have been far worse, since China would have had to hoard its supplies.

The United States actually had potential production capacity to make some medical supplies, such as high-quality masks. BARDA's leader, Bright, with help from industry leaders, had begun agitating about this issue in January. Beginning early in March, as emergency money finally began to flow, Kadlec, responsible for the Strategic National Stockpile, initiated a program that committed to buy hundreds of millions of N95 respirators, but the program had a timeline of a year and a half. Kushner's Project Airbridge had added emergency procurement of about 1.5 million N95s, but that was just a small fraction of what was needed.[21]

The U.S. government never really mounted a strong government N95 mask procurement program that could allow private firms to survive in a marketplace where the big buyers still preferred using their established, cheaper supply chains running back to China.

By early April, Kadlec had also assembled a program to buy hundreds of millions of more ordinary cloth masks. He worked with the underwear manufacturer Hanes. On April 2, Pence's chief of staff, Marc Short, took Kadlec's idea off the agenda of the task force, claiming concerns about funding. The plan for public distribution was dropped and many unused masks were handed out to whoever would take them. One of us saw them being worn by inmates in a Texas prison.[22]

The next day, as CDC announced its revised guidance on masks at a press conference, Trump, in attendance, stressed that the measure was voluntary and added: "I don't think I'm going to be doing it." Throughout the spring and summer, he was often seen and photographed at meetings, political rallies, and other events without a mask. He refused to wear a mask even when traveling in a state that required one, and often mocked those who wore them. Later, in October 2020, in an unforgettable moment of political theater, after he returned from Walter Reed Military Medical Center, where he had been hospitalized and treated for COVID-19, the president stood under the portico of the White House, in front of the television cameras, and ripped off his mask.[23]

By the time the first wave spread out around the country in the summer, about thirty states had mandated masks statewide in all indoor public spaces. Five states did not adopt mask mandates until much later, in November and December, during the pandemic's second wave. A dozen states never adopted broad indoor mask mandates, although some allowed local officials to mandate them.

Decisions about whether and when to mandate masks diverged sharply along political lines. Some Republican governors did mandate the use of masks, but those who did not were all Republicans. Not only were Democratic governors more likely than their Republican counterparts to mandate masks, but they were also more likely to mandate them early, before the arrival of the second wave in the late summer of 2020, and more likely to maintain these orders for a longer period of time.

This reluctance to require masks was fueled by politics. By the summer of 2020, many voters were angry and frustrated about the disruption they had experienced: shuttered businesses, closed schools, canceled gatherings, and the loss of friends and family members. In an election year, President Trump understood this anger and frustration and exploited it by, among other things, publicly opposing masks.

On July 20, 2020, as the first wave of the virus spread further around the country and the death toll mounted, the White House took another look at the mask issue. President Trump met with campaign advisers, studying polls showing his high disapproval rating. His pollster, Tony Fabrizio, and a campaign adviser, Jason Miller, told Trump that most Republicans—81 percent—actually supported some kind of mask requirement. The president could show leadership on this heading into the election.

Kushner agreed. He thought the move was a no-brainer. It would make people feel safer and ease tension. There were now plenty of masks available.

The chief of staff, Mark Meadows, knocked the idea down. "We can't do the masks," he said. "The base will just turn on you." President Trump agreed.[24]

In the face of public opposition from the leader of their own party, it was very difficult for state and local Republican officials to require masks. There were Republican governors who led on masking, including Asa Hutchinson of Arkansas, who said that a "mask was the uniform of a responsible citizen."[25]

But it was much easier to follow President Trump's lead by fighting against the use of masks, which some

Republicans did. In Georgia, the Republican governor refused to mandate the use of masks in his state. When the mayor of Atlanta, a Democrat, adopted a citywide mask mandate, he sued her for exceeding her authority. In Wisconsin, after the Democratic governor mandated the use of masks, the Republican-controlled legislature attempted to repeal the mandate and the Wisconsin Supreme Court ruled that the governor had exceeded his authority. In North Dakota, when the State Health Officer issued a statewide mask mandate, the Republican-controlled legislature passed a law prohibiting its enforcement. The Republican governor vetoed the legislation, but the state legislature overrode his veto.[26]

Lazar, who had participated in so many of these discussions, recalled: "I think masks became symbolic—and quite divergently so. For some, masks were symbolic of government gone wrong with overreach into personal decision space. For others they were a symbol that they cared about society and 'following the science.'"

The mask mandates, like the "hammer and dance" of lockdowns, were really symptoms of the deep problem. Without a more surgical toolkit, only blunt instruments were left.

One way to measure the U.S. problems with using effective toolkits is by noticing the deterioration of relative performance in comparison with the Europeans. During the first wave, in the spring and summer of 2020, the European performance, measured in excess mortality, was about 29 percent better. In the second wave, from October 2020 through the first half of 2021, this margin widened, to 51.5 percent. Little of this difference is probably related to vaccines. The United States actually had a brief head start in mass distribution of vaccines in the first half of 2021. The difference may have more relation to the accumulating divergence in quality of governance and the related politicization of public health.[27]

SURGICAL TOOLKITS TO REOPEN SCHOOLS

There were few issues in the Covid war that were more damaging and divisive than the battle over when and how to reopen schools. The first thing we can do is try to provide some comparative perspective. Below is a list of ten countries. For each, we provide the number of weeks that their schools were closed, or partly closed, to in-person instruction because of the pandemic during the first two years, from February 2020 to March 2022. They are listed from least closures to most. The data was collected by UNESCO, the education organization of the United Nations.[28]

France	2
Spain	15
United Kingdom	27
Israel	33
Denmark	35
Germany	38
Italy	38
Canada	52
United States	77
South Korea	79

A note about South Korea: South Korea, a society obsessed with education, has the most advanced educational technology setup in Asia, the region that has the most path-breaking educational technology in the world. Its ability to provide individualized remote learning is a generation ahead of what is available in almost all of the United States.

That may explain why South Koreans leaned on virtual or hybrid learning so much, though at great psychological and social cost. But what explains the United States?

One important distinction is simply the level of decision: the United States tends to have more local, decentralized school administration than is the case in most other countries. The initial decisions about school closures in the spring of 2020 were practically universal. No one knew for sure how dangerous the disease might be to children. Children are often the special prey of infectious diseases. As the spring passed and the demographic profile of COVID-19 vulnerability became clearer, two main concerns remained.

The first concern was that schools might become hot spots for contagion and community spread. The second concern was for the safety of the teachers, and their families. These concerns then had to be balanced with the many obvious costs to closing schools. The chart above gives a crude measure of how some different countries made those trade-offs.

During the fall of 2020, good studies were conducted to assess the danger of schools becoming hot spots for contagion. By January 2021, the results started coming in. On average, schools were not hot spots. Opening them did not affect community spread. People at schools were probably as safe, or safer, than they would be elsewhere.[29]

A stock explanation for why schools stayed closed more in the United States blamed teachers' unions. The unions were concerned about teacher safety. It was a reasonable concern. Teachers were anxious in other countries, too, like Germany.

The only good answer to these concerns was to adopt a toolkit of health measures that could make schools safer places to work. At least by late 2020, we think the case for reopening schools, aided by such toolkits, was getting stronger and stronger.

Here again, the Trump administration did not help. The president said schools should reopen, with little advice about how. The CDC's official position during the spring and summer of 2020 was to support reopening, but its successive, specific guidances during 2020 seemed all over the map and often impractical. There was little about ventilation and little about screening tests. Nor could the CDC make the risk-benefit trade-offs, since most of the wider social considerations were outside of its bailiwick.

During the 2020–21 academic year, many K-12 schools tried to reopen for in-person learning, then closed as the second wave of the virus swept the country during the fall months. Congress did not allocate substantial funds to aid school reopening until the end of 2020. School closures that fall of 2020 were common around the world, but in most other high-income countries authorities figured out a toolkit and reopened. That did not happen as much in the United States.

Closed schools, even with remote education, failed many students, particularly those already most at risk for disrupted learning. Most states allowed for some mix of virtual and limited in-person learning (the "hybrid" model) to protect particularly vulnerable students and families.[30]

During the 2020–21 school year, before vaccines became widely available, the toolkit to prevent Covid spread included designs that combined masking, hygiene, social distancing, smaller student cohorts, and improved ventilation. Such combinations could allow some methods to catch what others missed. Testing for COVID-19 could check how well the combinations were working and guide their use; and allow infected individuals and their direct contacts to isolate and quarantine. We offer two successful examples: one city program and one state program.

Texas schools reopened early in the fall of 2020. The city of San Antonio had a large Hispanic population in its schools, a population hit hard by COVID-19. Civic and business leaders in San Antonio decided to offer universal K-12 Covid testing at no cost to the schools. The state of Texas had a rapid antigen Covid testing program for K-12 schools, but it did not provide resources for testing every student.[31]

In San Antonio, a local charitable foundation paired with a blood bank to create a central Covid PCR testing lab (antigen tests were not yet readily available) that could combine samples (pooling) for efficiency and cost reduction, but also determine which individual in a pool was positive. Importantly, results were available within about twelve hours. That meant results were available before the start of school the next day. The foundation provided people to obtain samples, to ease the burden on school employees. They tested schools once per week.

Many schools in San Antonio and the surrounding districts participated, but the program was voluntary and not all schools participated. Once the pilot program was shown to work, state funds were added. San Antonio schools used a combination of methods to limit spread.

In the spring of 2021, the Commonwealth of Massachusetts created a statewide K-12 testing program to support reopening of its schools. The commonwealth also used PCR testing with rapid turnaround of less than twelve to twenty-four hours, also with pooling of samples, also free of charge to schools. Participation of schools was voluntary; parental consent for students was required.[32]

Massachusetts authorities created a network of preferred vendors for testing; the vendors provided both tests and staff. The world-class biotechnology base of the Boston-Cambridge region helped provide the system to report results and assess trends. The Broad Institute of MIT and Harvard hosted a regular forum of parents who shared experiences for how to get the job done. While not all districts and schools in the Commonwealth opted in, those that did got timely monitoring of Covid rates in their schools and data to support contact tracing.

In successful school testing programs, testing worked best when public-private partnerships helped the schools. Volunteers were important. Testing was expensive and had to be supported outside of traditional school budgets, and schools needed staffing help, too. Rapid results were necessary to provide timely information. With most school systems having local control, each district decided what to do. Teachers' unions were often uneasy about reopening schools until they felt assured that employees were safe or the district authorities forced the issue. A notable exception to this was New York City, which mandated random testing of all students in its schools.

Neither the CDC, nor anyone else, stepped up to do serious schoolwide studies of infection in schools. Daily testing of NBA players had, for instance, revealed incredible detail about risks and modes of transmission, as well as how to return safely to more crowded settings and which kinds of interventions worked best. No one did this sort of testing in schools, which should have happened during the fall of 2020.

At first, the Biden administration continued with the school position it had inherited—a general desire to reopen schools accompanied by a series of suggestions, many impractical, that allowed others to argue that standards of safety could not be met. Schools mainly stayed closed.

In the late spring of 2021, too late for the 2020–21 school year, again nonprofit efforts stepped in. They emphasized the emerging best practices, urging the new Biden administration to offer national leadership on how to reopen schools. Allen's group, working with the Covid Collaborative, Brown University's School of Public Health, and the New America Foundation, offered another road map (they had also offered a guide in December 2020).[33]

Again, the spring 2021 road map "was," Jeneen Interlandi wrote in the *New York Times Magazine*, "in short, everything that the CDC guidance was not. And it was the product of a strategy that felt obvious and simple: The task force engaged stakeholders in a sustained dialogue, incorporated input from schools and factored practical realities, like the need to move quickly, into its recommendations."[34]

By August 2021, the Biden administration had changed its tone and its guidance documents. It pressed hard to reopen schools during the 2021–22 school year. The guidance documents were revised, adding new material about ventilation and the use of screening tests. The administration had also helped enact legislation opening new spigots of money to help pay for such moves. At last, early in 2022, America's schools fully reopened for in-person instruction, for the first time in nearly two years.[35]

The toll on children from the failure in the United States to develop and implement a surgical toolkit for schools cannot be overstated. The impact on learning loss is increasingly being documented. Almost all children suffered important setbacks in skills development and knowledge but, predictably, children from disadvantaged communities as well as children with disabilities suffered the most. Virtual education and limited in-person learning (the "hybrid" model) did little to protect particularly vulnerable students, while imposing significant stress on families. American women, many leaving their jobs, disproportionately shouldered this burden. The U.S. Chamber of Commerce estimates that, over two years into the pandemic, an estimated one million women have still not returned to the workforce.[36]

Learning loss is, of course, only the most obvious way in which children were harmed in this pandemic. The deterioration in the mental health, but also the physical health, of children and adolescents is coming clearer into view. It is difficult to disentangle the role that school closures played in these harms; children were hardly immune to the economic losses, illnesses, and deaths of the adults around them. But one thing is clear: schools are much more than educational institutions. They are the physical spaces on which child and adolescent development critically depend. And when these buildings are shuttered, what is at stake is much more than what can be measured on standardized test scores.[37]

7

THE
HEALTHCARE
SYSTEM FRAYS

THE AMERICAN HEALTHCARE system is fragmented, organized into corporate systems fueled by a multi-party payer insurance system. Academic healthcare systems play another large part and county/city public hospitals often serve as a safety net.

Each hospital system makes its own decisions about how to allocate scarce resources. There is no formal mechanism for sharing space, staff, or supplies among hospitals within a region. Hospital systems have no incentive to share resources with their competitors. American healthcare economics disincentivize investment in preparedness.

As we explained in chapter 3, on the defenders in America, the public health departments are fundamentally detached from the healthcare system that developed during the twentieth century. To see what this means in practice, consider the federal government's program to fund emergency preparedness in the Hospital Preparedness Program.

Congress arranged the program so this money did not actually go to hospitals for preparedness. The money went primarily to state and local health departments.

Those departments could not "require" hospitals, or the healthcare system as a whole, to have some level of "preparedness." So, the public health departments had more or less free rein to do as they wished with this money.

Some kept the money to supplement the limited federal funds they receive for "public health emergency preparedness." Others offered money to hospital systems to encourage preparedness. Those that did give money to hospitals might have helped them a bit, but the amount of funding that any underfunded public health department could give to any hospital system was relatively insignificant. The program did not, and could not, require any particular level of hospital preparedness.

Even this program suffered cutbacks in the general neglect after the post-9/11 panic wore off. Many government leaders and elected officials assume that hospitals are flush with cash and that, once 9/11 fears faded, the private system should fund its preparedness. The reality is that the overwhelming majority of hospitals in the United States operate on thin margins. That is why large healthcare systems, seeing a chance to amass market power, are acquiring more and more hospitals and unaffiliated, independent, community hospitals are disappearing.

The large for-profit systems and the big nonprofit systems may make a huge amount of money, on the whole, and they use that to offset the costs of many smaller hospitals that bleed money every year. The big systems keep those smaller hospitals for strategic reasons—academic partnerships, deals with state lawmakers, or perhaps just the worthy desire to keep a community from being left in a healthcare desert. But the majority of systems are certainly not flush with cash for a rainy day. That, then, was the situation when the Covid war hit.

CODE BLUE FOR THE HEALTHCARE SYSTEM

The American healthcare system did not have the surge capacity to handle a major emergency. It still does not have it.

The enormous and very powerful HHS agency, the Centers for Medicare and Medicaid Services (CMS), took the step in 2017 of adding "Conditions of Participation" that required hospitals to meet some baseline level of preparedness. But the requirements were so rudimentary that they made little difference. To make a difference, CMS would have had to raise reimbursement rates to pump in more money so facilities would be ready for an emergency. Since there was no money, the unfunded mandates were understandably timid.

CMS has power to help build public health defenses. But it is not well linked to the executives forming strategy for national health security, who can link money to realistic peacetime defense requirements, set roles and missions for the defenders, and allocate public and private responsibilities. Absent such leadership, guidance, and resources, ultimate responsibility for preparedness is vague and the mandates are cosmetic, not worth the paper on which they are written.

The reality on the ground is that, for decades, hospital systems have tried to optimize staffing levels by downsizing and reengineering. This has led to repeated cycles of staffing shortages, particularly among nurses. Before the Covid war, industry experts were forecasting future shortages of doctors, nurses, and other healthcare personnel. When staffing shortages developed during past emergencies, like flu outbreaks or hurricanes, hospitals plugged local gaps by enlisting a ready (and expensive) reserve of traveling and per diem personnel. The per diem programs are stronger in bidding for nurses and respiratory therapists than in hiring physicians who provide emergency and critical care. The Covid pandemic created huge, sustained staffing gaps all over the country that could not be filled with such ad hoc reservists.

As we shift our focus from the people over to their equipment, we see the reality on the ground is that hospital systems increasingly use just-in-time inventory practices. They purchase their equipment and supplies through large group purchasing organizations. These organizations source nearly all PPE and most medical supplies and ventilators from other countries, especially China. In an emergency, they have no power over these foreign supply chains.

Reflecting to us about his work on the stockpile, a former HHS official concluded that shared responsibility is key. Not only does there need to be agreement at all levels about what to keep in the federal stockpile, but hospitals and health departments need to have plans and stockpiles of their own. Just-in-time supply chains aren't enough, and the federal stockpile can't be the only source of supplies in an emergency. In his view, "It's the SNS, not CVS."

The healthcare work force is poorly distributed. Healthcare workers and other resources are concentrated in major urban areas, but over 20 percent of the population resides far outside of these areas. Local hospitals in small towns and rural areas often lack equipment and adequately trained staff, and the nearest major medical center may be hundreds of miles away.

Many cities have some procedures and capability for handling a specific emergency, like a single mass casualty event. But a sustained war like this one went well beyond those plans. The better systems improvised, usually at the metro level, trying to pool and share resources, but with weak inventories of supplies and limited reserve capability to tap trained nurses and doctors. Small town, rural, and under-resourced communities were left to fend for themselves.

Once the pandemic arrived, a poorly prepared healthcare system quickly became a system in crisis.

This crisis immediately exposed the vulnerability of hospital supply chains. When Wuhan locked down, China limited exports of PPE and medical supplies. As the virus surged around the world, American hospitals tried to purchase more PPE, ventilators, and other supplies, but nothing was available. FEMA initiated Project Airbridge to move supplies from overseas, and the White House formed the Supply Chain Task Force, led by Kushner. A few domestic companies tried to enter the ventilator market. When shortages persisted, healthcare workers were forced to improvise by reusing disposable items, using garbage bags for gowns, wearing soiled N95s for weeks on end, and making homemade face shields.

With inadequate protection, healthcare workers were at grave risk. In the first year of the pandemic thirty-six hundred died from COVID-19. After the first wave of the virus crested, supplies improved gradually, but as the virus surged in subsequent waves, hospitals continued to experience episodic shortages. In our conversation with representatives of the American Nurses Association (ANA), we were told that the biggest issues facing nurses early in the pandemic could be summarized as "PPE, PPE, PPE, PPE."[1]

In another example of crisis improvisation, Lloyd Armbrust realized the need for domestically produced PPE capacity at the start of the pandemic and took it upon himself to help deliver. With a background in building companies, but knowing virtually nothing about mask production, Armbrust started Armbrust American in May 2020 and began building a factory in Texas that would eventually produce one million medical-grade masks and respirators per day, which he supplied to schools, medical professionals, businesses, and directly to the public.[2]

In our conversation with Armbrust, he emphasized his belief that such critical preparedness supplies need to have a domestic manufacturing base. He warned that domestic mask manufacturers struggle to compete with cheaper imports. His team demonstrated to one of us that Chinese masks and other PPE were often being sold for less than their estimated cost of production in China. These might be differences of only a few cents per mask but, to the large hospital buyers, that was enough to bypass domestic production. As the domestic producers then closed, the U.S. healthcare system remained reliant on foreign supply chains in a crisis.

This point was also made by economists and other experts who spoke with us. Absent guaranteed orders and other action from the U.S. government to pay for domestic preparedness, this cycle will continue.

This crisis also exposed the uneven distribution of hospital beds from one community to the next. In its early days, the pandemic overwhelmed hospitals in New York City and several other cities on the East Coast.

Later, in the summer and fall of 2020, as Covid hot spots popped up around the country, many rural hospitals were simply overwhelmed. Doctors managed heavy caseloads in makeshift ICUs, running from code to code, day after day. Patients died in hallways. Many of these communities suffered high fatality rates, sometimes fivefold the rates seen in well-resourced, less-stressed communities.

Many rural hospitals ran out of ICU beds. Usually, within the region, others had excess capacity. But because hospital systems were not required, incentivized, or used to sharing the load, they were forced to go it alone. They had to find available beds for their transfer patients with limited or zero awareness of capacity within the region. Unable to expand their supply of ICU beds quickly, they restricted demand instead by cancelling elective surgeries.

Notice again the missing institutions that could provide an organized common defense. During the Covid war, some states and regions stepped up. They improvised what needed to be done. Sometimes this happened through voluntary cooperation. In Massachusetts, particularly in Boston, hospital leaders created groups of what one observer, Paul Biddinger, called "capacity specialists" from competing hospitals. They talked about which hospitals were overloaded and who had capacity. "Managing as a community," Biddinger told us, meant they never ran out of ICU beds or ventilators. One of us who worked on these problems in the federal government, listening to this, commented that "Biddinger is describing how things should be done, but it wasn't done like that everywhere."

In some states, governors used executive orders. Many states, such as Minnesota and Arizona, ended up doing excellent work, making up protocols for how to share patient loads and coordinate healthcare service. Once the executive orders expired, though, the improvisations faded. Hospital executives would not do these things voluntarily and CMS did not set standards to require regular peacetime coordination unless an emergency had been declared.

The healthcare system was the final line of defense against the pandemic. As it frayed and sometimes failed, healthcare workers, especially those on the front line, paid a huge price.

Before COVID-19 arrived, clinicians were already in a crisis of burnout. Their working conditions were increasingly difficult, with less autonomy, the constant drudgery of maintaining electronic health records, and other ballooning administrative burdens. When the pandemic arrived, these already depleted workers were strained ever further, especially those on the front line, who worked long hours in chaotic conditions with inadequate PPE. There was no vaccine in the first year. Some sickened; some died. Exhausted and fearing for their own safety, they suffered anxiety, depression, and emotional distress.

By the beginning of 2022, more than 60 percent of physicians were reporting symptoms of burnout, which one healthcare leader called "the biggest increase of emotional exhaustion that I've ever seen, anywhere in the literature." Constantly worrying that they might expose their friends and families to COVID-19, many caregivers isolated themselves. They stripped and showered in their front yards, stopped hugging their families, or completely stayed away from home after shifts, further straining their mental health. The camaraderie they had with each other eroded over time with isolation, elimination of social events, and the constant need to wear PPE. All this then mixed into a medical culture that was highly perfectionist and stigmatized mental illness. Many just suffered in silence.[3]

In the first year of the pandemic one in five healthcare workers resigned, retired, or were fired. In 2022, 44 percent of infectious disease fellowship slots for young physicians went unfilled. As one specialist explained to us, a doctor-in-training "could take care of sick Covid in the ICU and get paid ICU money, or I could get death threats in [infectious disease] and not pay back my student loans."

Throughout the pandemic, many hospitals reported critical staff shortages. Hospitals responded to these shortages, as they always had, by hiring traveling workers. When states hit hardest by the virus offered high salaries and lucrative bonuses, many healthcare workers relocated, leaving many poorer hospitals even more short-staffed. Immigration and travel constraints made it harder for firms to recruit foreign residents or nurses.[4]

Most states have Crisis Standard of Care (CSC) plans allowing hospitals to triage scarce resources once the state formally declares a crisis, but only a few states made formal CSC declarations. Some states ignored their plans, and sometimes the chaotic conditions in hospitals made it difficult for a state to determine whether a crisis had begun for a particular resource in a particular geographic area. In many hospitals, individual healthcare workers were forced to make difficult triage decisions anyway, sometimes without the necessary training, guidance, or legal protections.

During the crisis, community-based care providers also struggled. Overnight, the demand for outpatient services plummeted, as patients canceled in-person appointments. Fewer appointments meant less revenue, and providers responded by laying off staff and reducing services. Some closed their doors. Most providers pivoted to telehealth, which slowly gained acceptance among patients, but one study estimated that half of all Americans lacked access to high-speed internet at home.

As the final wall of defense crumbled or, in some places, collapsed, healthcare providers fell back on battlefield-style triage. The thousands of nurse, doctor, respiratory therapist, and paramedic survivors of the Covid frontline battlefields still carry many scars.

Healthcare workers have mixed feelings about military metaphors like these. For some, they ring true. For others, it can make them uncomfortable. While there are certainly similarities between doctors and soldiers in this context, there are also important differences. For example, unlike soldiers, clinicians felt they never signed up to risk their lives. Many viewed medicine as a job, more than a calling, and were not interested in making greater than ordinary sacrifices for that job, even though many did.

The military consciously builds camaraderie and offers respites from the front lines. Covid undermined camaraderie in hospitals and left workers little respite. Further, some felt the war/hero narrative was used by hospital executives as a way of evading accountability for the burdens and sacrifices of employees (e.g., send a "hero" email to the entire hospital to distract from botched communication or lack of PPE).

BIOMEDICAL SURVEILLANCE— ONE MORE CUT

In chapter 4, on containment, we introduced the issue of biomedical surveillance in the United States, getting data from healthcare facilities. There we treated it as a kind of early warning system.

We returned to the issue again in chapter 6, on the tools for community defense. There we emphasized what communities could learn about who was at risk and what tools might work.

We come back to this issue again in this chapter, on healthcare. Here we see it as a way to monitor and coordinate the capacity to deliver services, pool supplies, and see what kind of care works best.

As we pointed out earlier, private healthcare organizations often have very good information on what is going on in their facilities and with their patients. Some have data insight tools that provide remarkable and up-to-date information. Companies are understandably reluctant to share those revealing dashboards, some quite advanced, either with their competitors or with the government, especially in a situation where they get no useful information or support in return. They might, however, support a national approach that helps everyone understand threatening conditions. Medicare and Medicaid, through CMS, have some potential regulatory tools.

This is an interesting opportunity. It is not unique to healthcare. The airline industry, for instance, has a system it calls Aviation Safety Information Analysis and Sharing (ASIAS) that allows companies to share information about incidents with a third party, in this case, the MITRE Corporation, which employs thousands of people, has extensive data handling capabilities, and works with the Federal Aviation Administration. The electric utility industry also uses a third party, the North American Electric Reliability Corporation (NERC), to help regulate the power grid, working with the Department of Energy. In cybersecurity, the Department of Homeland Security convenes "industry specific" analysis centers to pool information.

There is an emerging consensus in the healthcare industry that necessary data sharing in the United States can no longer be strictly voluntary, hit or miss. The movement to electronic health records offers an opportunity. Healthcare providers badly want accurate, actionable data on health threats. As we write this, in early 2023, they are anxious about capacity and trends in a challenging health season that combines renewed outbreaks of Covid, RSV (respiratory syncytial virus), flu, and more.

Privacy has to be protected and companies will also have concerns about tort liability. If the system is designed well, focused on public health dangers, this is a solvable problem. A changing CDC does have a role it can play, including with its new Center for Forecasting and Outbreak Analytics.

APPLYING BEST PRACTICES?

When nurses and doctors provided face-to-face (mask-to-mask) care for their individual patients, they were not implementing coordinated public health strategies for healthcare delivery. There were no best treatment practices to review or share. They MacGyvered their way through it.

The CDC's limited biomedical surveillance effort did not provide this guidance because it did not quickly link confirmed Covid cases to the clinical information about the patients. The data did not show what kinds of people were most in danger, or what kinds of people were being helped by treatments. The CDC was not itself really at fault; CDC collects no data on its own. It relies completely on its state and local partners. Practitioners had to wait until academic researchers or better-informed foreign governments could offer such insight.

Individual hospitals or healthcare companies might have better records. But their data is not connected enough to provide wider insight. In a crisis, that problem makes it difficult for leaders to investigate, on a large scale, what is working and not working. It is hard to learn and implement lessons.

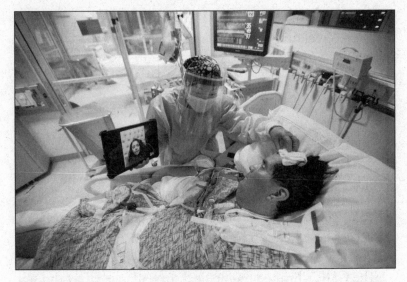

Registered Nurse Kat Yi holds an iPad up to Eduardo Rojas, who is inside the ICU at Providence St. Jude Medical Center in Fullerton, California, so that he can talk to his wife on Christmas Day 2020. Because of measures to prevent coronavirus infection, seriously ill patients were often isolated and hospital staff had to serve as a link between them and their family members. PHOTO CREDIT: FRANCINE ORR/LOS ANGELES TIMES VIA GETTY IMAGES

It was, for instance, a stroke of luck that doctors began informally sharing the news that high-flow nasal cannulas (thin tubes) were working as well for delivering oxygen to their patients as ventilators. This was a huge insight: high-flow patients could be managed awake in a standard hospital floor bed, while patients on ventilators required deep sedation in ICUs. Physicians now had another tool in their box to care for the overwhelming load of critically ill patients in their hospitals.

There was similar early luck in the revival and repurposing of "proning" (turning patients from their backs to their stomachs) for critically ill patients. This salvage method rapidly spread across the world through informal communication before it could be formally tested in trials. Proning is difficult. It requires a team of at least five to seven care providers to gown and mask, then lift and turn, without dislodging tubes and IV lines. But with little else to offer the sickest of the sick Covid patients, proning became a rite of passage, an expression that they were doing everything they could to honor their commitment to saving lives.

These were anecdotal observations, not the product of systematic data analysis, which—even to use data that "deidentified" patients—was beyond the capacity of the healthcare system at the beginning of the 2020s. In chapter 9, on medical countermeasures and drugs, we note that Britain had a system that could enable such analysis, and that their system, and the scientists using it, yielded one of the most important treatment breakthroughs in the crisis. We believe such a biomedical surveillance system can be adopted in America.

In addition to a better system of biomedical surveillance gathering data on what works, why not help doctors just share their best practices? The Covid war again reveals possibilities for how to do better. The doctors in the field, treating patients, naturally learned a lot and shared what they learned. But translating what they learned into broad formal guidance was slow, lagging months behind what was already happening in the field.

For example, monoclonal antibodies became a valuable treatment. But the treatments became less useful as new variants of the virus escaped these agents. Physicians needed to learn about this quickly.

In our vision of a national health security enterprise, with strategic-level governance, leaders might get frequent insight from an organized network of advisers, conducting weekly or even daily conference calls to update each other and plugged into the data gathering we also recommend. Best would be advisers working at institutions that handle large numbers of patients and have the capability to conduct rigorous clinical research on infectious disease. Such networks already exist in the Infectious Diseases Society of America and more informally. Each part of the nation has such hospitals. Also valuable would be health systems that routinely track the patients "longitudinally," not just services that hospitals provided.

Our healthcare organizations don't always do a great job of translating possibility (new drugs, tests, or treatments) into actual practice by physicians in the field. That has been, and still is, a large problem in the Covid war. Americans have been learning how to do better. It is time to translate what they have learned into enduring lessons.

8

TRUST AND CONFIDENCE BREAK DOWN

A NYONE FAMILIAR WITH the history of public health interventions in America knows that they have often been resented and sometimes fiercely resisted. They have been seen as infringing on individual liberties or as unjustly targeting marginal and powerless communities regarded as unhealthy sources of disease. Yet many of these public health interventions were vitally successful. They made America's growing cities much safer places in which to live.

The American healthcare system has a unique, distinctive history, different from systems found in most other developed countries. When the Covid invasion hit, many Americans entered the crisis with a reasonably positive attitude toward medical professionals and their personal healthcare providers. They knew how to ask for help and believed that they had a good chance of readily getting it. Many less affluent rural and urban Americans, though, had long seen the healthcare system as remote, alien, and distrusted.

The roots of distrust go deep among communities that have long felt marginalized. They include the legacy of the Tuskegee Study, in which Public Health Service doctors ran a study that, for decades, failed to treat syphilis in black males in order to study what happened to them. The cultural memory in the black community of this episode, which ended with press disclosures in 1972, is profound.[1]

There is a fundamental tension in American society, as in other countries, between individual freedom and collective responsibility. There is no simple solution to this tension. The tension can be mitigated by hyper-local efforts that connect everyday healthcare advice to more individuals in a trusted way.

People have to experience the public health system more as positive help than negative confinement. It helps them stay safe as they go about their lives. It helps them find healthcare. Other developed countries have bridged this gap with outreach like that provided by public health nurses and other community health workers who do home visits and outreach in schools and neighborhood centers. Such outreach can connect ordinary people with the public health and healthcare system, building their trust and earning their confidence.

Not only did the United States lack the public health workforce needed to connect with the community and help them cope with a pandemic, but also it lacked situation awareness about the needs and resources in many communities. Leaders therefore often had little idea how Americans would respond to their health initiatives, or what they might do on their own, if asked.

Thus, the United States entered the pandemic crisis with weak surge capacity to reach local communities and limited public trust. The public health community had long expected that such a situation might produce a crisis of confidence in public and private institutions. Their worst fears were realized.[2]

AN UNPRECEDENTED EXPERIMENT

Ignorant about their public health institutions and detached from many community health concerns, American leaders entering the Covid war plunged ahead with a breathtaking political and social experiment. Facing a dangerous pandemic, they adopted the broadest, most ambitious, and intrusive set of government controls on social behavior in the history of the United States.

Given the lack of preparation at all levels of government, mistakes were inevitable and to be expected, perhaps even excusable. Public confidence never recovered entirely from the April 2020 flip-flop about the usefulness of face masks. Anyone who had studied the work that had been done about how to communicate with people about risk and do public outreach could have anticipated the ensuing confused, frustrated, and hostile responses.[3]

Sadly, public communication did not get any better during the late spring and summer of 2020. That was the time when national authorities might have caught their breath, gathered evidence, made plans, and networked with organizations that had better roots in communities across America.

For example, looking ahead to the problem of distributing vaccines, a National Academy of Sciences committee, co-chaired by William Foege and Helene Gayle, issued a report at the beginning of October 2020 that stressed how important it was for the CDC to develop a campaign using proven techniques from risk and health communication, social marketing, and behavioral science. The committee warned that the government—probably CDC and FDA working together, perhaps with Operation Warp Speed—would also need to build a risk communication and community engagement program that would partner with hospitals, pharmacies, faith-based organizations, community centers, schools, and universities to refine what to say, listen to reactions, and adjust. That didn't happen.[4]

All levels of American government started with a finite amount of social capital, which determined what people were willing to accept, and for how long. In order to preserve and increase that capital, governments needed to help the public to make a seemingly endless series of fateful choices, sometimes framed as if they were between "your money or your life." We have explained why we think this binary framing was false and tragically unnecessary.

These were complex decisions, made under difficult circumstances, with incomplete information. In addition, these were not one-time decisions, but decisions that communities were forced to revisit again and again, as the virus surged and receded in different parts of the country.

As tools to reopen, like rapid antigen tests, became available, by the fall of 2020, the deeper problem was that state and local authorities still lacked adequate guidance on how to assemble and use those tools to reopen safely and manage

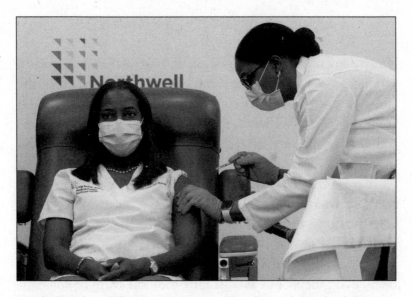

Sandra Lindsay, left, a nurse at Long Island Jewish Medical Center in Queens, New York, receives a dose of the Pfizer-BioNTech COVID-19 vaccine on December 14, 2020. She was the first person in the United States to receive a Covid vaccination outside of clinical trials. PHOTO CREDIT: MARK LENNIHAN/GETTY IMAGES

the risks to their communities. Policy became paralyzed, especially with school closures.[5]

. As this false and unnecessary public framing took hold, some state legislatures curtailed the emergency powers of their governors and health departments, convinced that their actions were dangerous and irresponsible abuses of authority. We discussed how masks became a continuing flashpoint. Following President Trump's lead, many Republican governors refused to adopt mask mandates or prohibited local governments and private businesses from mandating the use of masks.

AGGRAVATING POLARIZATION

We have criticized the quality of practical public health guidance, including guidance on how to reopen during the summer and fall of 2020, including the guidance offered from the CDC. We have commented on the improvisations, some of them quite remarkable, among many state and local defenders.

It is therefore only fair to also note the unique environment in which these beleaguered public health authorities were working during those months. By May 2020 and on through the rest of the year, President Trump and some of his key advisers were effectively at war with much of their own government. The war usually took the form of constant public sniping, above all from the president. Behind the scenes, this warfare took the form of constant efforts to muffle, delay, or critique public guidance.

We would find these interventions more understandable if they were part of a constructive dialogue to make the guidances more workable and practical. Close examination of what happened, revealed for instance in reports of the House Select Subcommittee on the Coronavirus Crisis, does not show such a story. These were not interventions to devise practical toolkits of the kind we have discussed. They instead were efforts to downplay the gravity of the crisis, limit the breadth of testing, or promote ideas that, somehow, the elderly could practically be segregated from otherwise unhindered community spread, perhaps with the hope of attaining the tempting mirage of "herd immunity."

Public health and hospital workers received death threats. Many resigned, retired, or were fired. Already understaffed public health departments could not fill open positions, leaving them even less prepared for the next pandemic.

As President Trump gave up on crisis management during April and May 2020 and returned to wishing the crisis away, he capitalized on the predictable lockdown fatigue and resentment. President Trump poured acid on the strained bonds holding together the disparate communities that were already experiencing the crisis in such different ways.

Without effective national leadership, everyone was on their own, turning to social media for arguments and reinforcement, fanning resentment and fatigue. Parents had to figure out whether and how to send kids to schools. Schools had to figure out under what conditions to let students into buildings or let them play. Those with different opinions were left to fight it out. Such fights moved into workplaces, nursing homes, stores, and restaurants.

THE RISE OF MISINFORMATION
AND DISINFORMATION

This political and social situation was a petri dish for pathological social media. The Covid war was the first national emergency to unfold against the background of the fragmented twenty-first-century information universe, channeled in social networks that massively profited from amplifying hate and bile. To that toxic environment, add high-level public confusion, the constant spray of presidential acid, and substantial Russian and Chinese cyber mischief-making.

Misinformation spread like wildfire, some of it truly fantastical in nature. By mid-2021, Facebook and Instagram had removed some 18 million COVID-19 posts as potentially dangerous misinformation and labeled over 167 million posts as containing false statements. Some came from the misinformed, some from those seeking political, financial, or other personal ends. More sophisticated disinformation sowed doubt about the value of masks, the side effects of vaccines, and the benefits of quack cures. Vaccines were pronounced ineffective even though there was clear and resounding evidence to the contrary. In both the Delta (2021) and Omicron (2021–22) waves, the vast majority of hospitalized patients were unvaccinated.[6]

Foreign sources of disinformation engaged and surreptitiously influenced topics such as viral origin and vaccine quality using coordinated disinformation campaigns. These malicious actors took advantage of social media platforms to exploit and aggravate the preexisting fault lines in American society.

This was the first national experience where every citizen virtually every day was confronted by a torrent of misinformation. Beginning with Russian campaigns targeting the 2016 U.S. elections, Americans were confronting a cascade of disinformation the magnitude of which was only gradually appreciated. There were earnest attempts to counter this, but the traditional government channels of press conferences and traditional media outlets were not adequate to the task, as research has shown. And when government itself mumbled or misinformed, it invited derision.

Policymakers could have gathered the information that people most need, tested messages to ensure that they would be understood as intended, disseminated them through popular channels, partnered with trusted intermediaries, monitored how things were going, and changed course as needed. Instead, they improvised. Often they sent untested, incoherent, uncoordinated messages, and then deplored the public confusion that this caused.[7]

Under difficult circumstances, West Virginia made an effort to provide clear and practical communication. Its leaders thought hard about what their people wanted to know and how best to present it to them.[8]

People felt entitled to get answers to serious questions. They rightfully demanded transparency. Why were there lockdowns in places with no observed disease? What was wrong with walking on the beach during lockdowns? When was cleaning surfaces just "hygiene theater"? How could the bivalent booster be approved without human tests? Something was wrong, if the explanations were not forthcoming. Capable political leaders do not usually handle the communications surrounding their major policy initiatives in such a slipshod way.

CRISIS MANAGEMENT AS
A VITAL POLITICAL PROCESS

As we pointed out in chapter 6, on community defense with few tools, there were many improvised efforts to create crisis management processes. Some of these efforts paid off in higher-quality policies with good links to what was happening in the field, in the clinics or emergency rooms, with practical knowledge about workplaces or schools, and links to people or institutions who could get things done out in neighborhoods.

What we wish to stress here is that, where the improvised crisis management efforts worked, *they also helped politically.* They mattered not just because they might make policymakers a little wiser. They mattered because, if the process worked, people felt heard and understood.

That is because the toolkit must include crisis communication. The toolkit would include procedures for gathering and analyzing real-time data, monitoring the state of the pandemic, in order to inform the public and see how the public responded. The toolkit would not rely on the *Atlantic* magazine or the *New York Times* or the Johns Hopkins Center for Health Security to organize ad hoc public information about the development of the crisis.

These processes cannot be built from the top down. They need to build up from public-private partnerships that engage local messengers who have earned some trust in the community. For example, by September 2021, as Covid rates in rural America were more than 50 percent higher than anywhere else in the country, the Covid Collaborative and the Ad Council worked to build up a ground game, working with partners like the American Farm Bureau Federation, the Cooperative Extension System, and others to provide more trusted outreach in five states—Tennessee, Arkansas, Texas, Florida, and Minnesota—in areas with especially low vaccination rates.[9]

There were successes. Some American Indian communities achieved high immunization rates, using their tribal sovereignty to create plans that worked in their communities, including reliance on networks of community health workers.[10]

However, such successes were not systematically documented and shared, nor were the many failures. As a result, America's national learning curve through 2020 and on into 2021 was flat or even negative.

Because authorities were flying blind about how the virus was spreading, many communities probably imposed social controls long before they needed to. One of us analogizes such controls to a fire extinguisher. It is best against a small fire. Use it before a fire and it runs out. But it cannot put out a large fire. Timing was hard when authorities could not track the virus spread. So they used up a lot of their social capital before their crisis really arrived.

Other communities, like Austin, Texas, used local experts to develop their own metrics for controls—a transparent stoplight chart that went up and down as cases surfaced, and which people could understand, to guide the "hammer and dance" cycle we have already described. In other words, part of a high-quality policy was also the way, using a reasonable communication plan, the policy shared high-quality understanding of what was going on—earning trust and confidence.

Public health experts knew that a pandemic was coming, and another after that, even if they could not predict the details. They knew that governing authorities needed a toolkit in place, come what may, that could maximize safety and minimize controls. We discussed that in the previous chapter.

And such a toolkit would include prototype public messages, tested to see if people found them credible and understandable, adaptable to emergency conditions. It would include connections with community partners, with the training and resources to go the last mile to deliver messages, hear concerns, and relay them to local and national authorities.

Some public health experts understood much of this. They knew they would need to explain the risks, benefits, and priorities for vaccines and treatments. They knew they would have to deal with distrust and disinformation, while also protecting the most vulnerable groups. Operating in a system designed for another age, already struggling to meet even their existing responsibilities, they lacked the capacity to grapple with these new tasks.

The value of these innovations is not just in policy; it is in politics. Different stakeholders are included. Their points of view are welcomed. A lot more people then understand what is happening and why, which earns trust and confidence.

A STRATEGY FOR VACCINE ACCEPTANCE?

During 2021, after the vaccines arrived, the strategic opportunity changed. A fortuitous combination of long-term investment in basic research, enterprising scientists, private companies, and government entrepreneurs had developed effective vaccines and started up very large production lines.

Lots of vaccine, but only a sketchy distribution plan, one that delivered to states but left open many last-mile distribution issues in the hands of state and local authorities. Partly because of the Trump administration's own ambivalent message about the crisis, a massive public campaign to explain and promote the vaccines had not been prepared.

Getting vaccines into the appropriate arms requires logistical support and willing recipients. The Operation Warp Speed planners, who did many things well, did little to bring vaccines and people together. The program had none of the behavioral science expertise needed to take full advantage of the biomedical and manufacturing capabilities it had assembled.

Though proudly touting its role in developing the vaccines, the Trump administration was ambivalent in recommending their use. So, little was done to communicate about vaccine risks and benefits in a clear and understandable way, based on the clinical trials and subsequent experience with vastly larger groups of people.

Again, nonprofits tried to fill the void. The Covid Collaborative and the Ad Council stepped up to create a $250 million vaccine education campaign, one of the larger public education campaigns in U.S. history. But it was not enough.[11]

The new Biden administration, for the first time, created a functional day-to-day crisis management structure in the White House. It also announced a comprehensive national Covid response plan, something the previous administration had not articulated. These were important and positive achievements. However, taking over an improvised set of arrangements, the new team struggled to explain its actions, leaving the public further behind.[12]

That was the situation in the first half of 2021, when the Biden administration faced strategic choices about whether or how to mandate vaccines. It had to decide whether to go all in on mandating vaccines, up to the limits of its formal and informal authority. It had to make that choice soon enough to be ready for the time, by the summer of 2021, when vaccine production would hit full industrial scale and the large-scale evidence would be available to replace emergency use authorization with a mandate.

Vaccine skepticism and pandemic fatigue were certainly no surprise. Surveys in the fall of 2020 were showing that 30–40 percent of adults did not want to take the vaccine. Black Americans and Latinos were particularly vaccine hesitant.[13]

Vaccine mandates adopted in 2021 by governments or by private companies met legal and legislative challengers. Hundreds of lawsuits were litigated during 2021 and 2022. That process continues. Some states adopted vaccine mandates; some states attempted to ban their use. Well-crafted vaccine mandates by private employers were usually upheld by the courts.

In the summer and fall of 2021, the Biden administration chose to mandate vaccines about as far as it could, testing the limits of federal executive authority. The administration first mandated "vaccination or test" (frequent testing if the person was exempt from the mandate) for federal employees and contractors. This mandate was generally upheld but, in August 2022, the administration chose to suspend it.

Also, in the summer and fall of 2021, the administration used CMS rules to mandate vaccination of most healthcare workers. The Supreme Court found that HHS had the authority to do this.

Finally, the administration's Labor Department tried to adopt a vaccine mandate for all workplaces with more than a hundred employees. There the Supreme Court found that the administration had gone too far. It reversed this effort to address public health through a broad occupational health regulation.[14]

The administration's decisions to push vaccine mandates may have reflected a pessimistic assessment of the administration's ability to influence the American public. Maybe it judged that a more effective public campaign of persuasion was too difficult, given the way polarization had primed vaccination campaigns to falter in Republican areas.

Trump had been vaccinated. In April 2021 he told two reporters, Peter Baker and Susan Glasser, that the administration had asked him to tape a public service announcement urging Americans to get their shots. "They want me to do a commercial," he told them, "because it seems that a lot of people that are inclined to be with me don't like the concept of—you know, they're antivax." He said the government had asked him and he was considering it.[15]

At an Alabama rally in August, Trump said, "I recommend take the vaccines. I did it. It's good. Take the vaccines." His audience booed. And that was that.

Interviewing Trump again a few months later, in November 2021, Baker and Glasser asked about that public service ad. Why hadn't he made the ad? "They [the Biden administration] have not asked me," he replied. They reminded him that he was the one who said the government had asked him to do it.

"Not that I know of, no," he answered.

Democratic areas did end up with high vaccination rates. In a July 2022 survey, 90 percent of Democrats reported some level of vaccination compared to 69 percent of Republicans.[16]

The Biden team did create innovative and successful programs to boost vaccine uptake in black, Hispanic, and American Indian communities, where vaccine acceptance was so doubtful. In the spring of 2021, white Americans were significantly more likely to have been vaccinated than black or Hispanic Americans. That turned around. By late 2021, the Hispanic vaccination rate was higher than the white rate, and the black rate was almost as high. As a result, the racial gap in death rates had also disappeared. This disappearance was a remarkable achievement, a tribute to passionate advocacy and hard work by health officials at all levels of American government. They used the emerging playbook on working with respected community leaders for better communication and building trust—and it worked.[17]

Yet, by the time the supply of vaccines was abundant, with vaccines available on demand, the general demand had weakened. Skeptics were winning increasing market share. Take-up of booster vaccines also faltered.

Going back again to comparing the EU and U.S. mortality numbers, it is striking to compare performance in the second half of 2021. During the second wave of the virus, from the last quarter of 2020 through the first half of 2021, the European excess mortality rate was 51.5 percent lower than in the United States. During the second half of 2021 this difference widened to 83 percent. Yet in 2021 the Americans had access to more vaccine doses, sooner, than the Europeans did.[18]

At this stage, a fundamental difference was vaccine uptake. That difference emerged clearly during the second half of 2021. It continued throughout 2022. Studies, including one co-authored by a member of this group, suggest that by early 2022 the cost of this difference, in American lives lost, was already in the range of between 120,000 and more than 350,000 excess deaths. [19]

Almost all adult Americans eventually did get vaccinated, at least once. They were, however, slower to do it and less likely to get needed booster shots.[20]

The essence of strategy is to concentrate available means for maximum effect at minimum cost. The vaccines were the strategic power drive in this war. The problems in communication that began in 2020 and the associated political polarization can indeed be called toxic. The substantial difference in death rates after vaccines became readily available, between the United States and other high-income countries, is one way to measure the toll.

9

FIGHTING BACK
WITH DRUGS
AND VACCINES

I N A MODERN war, as defenders muster their arsenal of
weapons, they have to decide which weapons work best.
They have to buy, build, and deploy them. They have to learn
how to use them effectively in practice. All this has to be
knitted together in a strategy, using the different forces and
their weapons.

In the Covid war, it was hard to decide which weapons
worked best. None worked all that well, at least at first, and
American evaluations of them were thrown off by damaging
political interference. In the one weapons-selection process
sheltered from that interference, vaccines emerged as a powerful weapon but the normal U.S. government processes
could not buy, build, and deploy them. Public sector innovation and private sector ingenuity came to the rescue. The
drugs and vaccines that were developed were never knitted
well into strategies for their best possible employment in the
field.

EVALUATING THE WEAPONS

Remember that, in the 2019 Crimson Contagion exercise, the antiviral medicine (for a flu virus) was assumed to be already there. In 2020, when Covid hit, the few broad spectrum antiviral medicines already on the table did not help much.

When Covid hit, the defenders had to judge which weapons might work best. There has been no modern war in which heads of state, or their non-expert staff, have intervened usefully to direct which missile or tank would work best. Such leaders can set priorities. They can pick capable people. They can encourage promising experiments, even unorthodox ones. They don't do well when they try to judge, or prejudge, the results of those experiments in the air, at sea, or on the ground.

In the Covid war, those experiments had to be evaluated by scientists, statisticians, biomedical engineers, doctors, and nurses. Developing weapons involves medical imagination and experimentation, from theory to laboratory to animal studies and then clinical trials on human beings. Approved medical countermeasures are often quickly used in practice. They are put into people's bodies in the millions, or even billions.

A good process required setting up institutions to identify research participants and run trials rapidly, if necessary on a large scale, to evaluate a number of promising drugs. That evaluation had to be scientific and clinical. It had to be independent of the people pitching the products.

For the U.S. government, the main evaluators in HHS were the research leaders (NIH: Collins and Fauci); the development leaders (BARDA: first Bright, succeeded by

Gary Disbrow working for the ASPR, Kadlec); and the regulators (FDA, headed by Stephen Hahn; and the directors of his centers for drugs, Janet Woodcock, and for biologics/vaccines, Peter Marks).

BARDA, the Biomedical Advanced Research and Development Authority, had an annual budget before the Covid war of about $1.5 billion. BARDA had funded development of an Ebola vaccine. That vaccine missed the 2014–15 outbreak but was ready in time for another local outbreak that happened in Africa in 2018–19.[1]

The Pentagon also developed medical defenses against an enemy biological attack. It focused more on countering biological agents that were known to be usable as weapons, like anthrax. In January 2020, Pentagon leaders told their biodefense officials that the Covid crisis was a civilian matter, to be left with those agencies. The Pentagon thus stayed on the sidelines of the fight for months, until Secretary of Defense Mark Esper offered to help with the vaccines push.

For any of these evaluators, a crucial, unglamorous, task was the enormously complex arrangement of human clinical trials to prove safety and effectiveness. These are the tests to find out if weapons work.

If the institutions are in place, an epidemic can make it easier to conduct trials, since so many people are getting sick. In a crisis, such trials can be accomplished in a few weeks—if the institutions are in place.

The British government has recently issued a technical report on its lessons learned in the Covid war. One of the striking features of this report is how well British officials and scientists used their institutions, and their databases, and adapted them during the crisis to run trials and gain rapid feedback. The British setup provided insights that probably saved many thousands of lives, possibly even that of President Trump himself.[2]

Doctors and nurses confronting the first wave soon felt they were in a battle zone, with too little they could do, including the challenge of just protecting themselves from infection. They tried different ways to give patients oxygen and oxygenate their blood. They tried anti-inflammatory medicines to ease the body's reaction to the virus.

During the summer of 2020, these desperate doctors got some help. The system in the United Kingdom produced an excellent analysis of COVID-19 treatment alternatives. Scientists at Oxford University, Martin Landray and Peter Horby, used their country's system to conduct clinical trials on a large scale under emergency conditions, with help from a major foundation, the Wellcome Trust.

In June 2020, the British trial, called Recovery, showed that a powerful immunosuppressive steroid, dexamethasone, dramatically reduced the death rate of hospitalized patients requiring oxygen support or mechanical ventilation. It could cut the chance of death among those sickest patients by as much as a third.[3]

This British work would go on to save a great many lives. Dexamethasone was widely available and cheap, though shortages soon cropped up.

When COVID-19 hit, the best labs in America studying coronaviruses were led by Ralph Baric (University of North Carolina) and Mark Denison (Vanderbilt University). Baric and Denison then thought the most promising antivirals for COVID-19 might be remdesivir, made by Gilead, and something then called EIDD-2801, later called molnupiravir.

Remdesivir had a safety track record because it had been used against Ebola. But the drug was unwieldy because it had to be delivered with an IV infusion for thirty minutes to two hours. It was also very expensive.

A part of the NIH, led by Cliff Lane, tried to quickly set up a system of emergency clinical trials in the United States. The WHO made a similar effort. But those trials struggled to get enough participants. Until 2022, the United States was not able to create a system that could test existing, repurposed drugs as definitively as the Recovery program did in Britain. Those weaknesses, and the lack of data, set the stage for the fights over drug approvals during 2020.

The NIH and WHO trials did confirm some limited value for remdesivir; the FDA gave remdesivir an emergency use authorization in May 2020. It had modest value in helping some patients recover more quickly. A Chinese study seemed to show no effect. The drug continued to be prescribed in the hope that it could have some benefit for certain patients.[4]

Molnupiravir had been developed by a company called Ridgeback. The safety of EIDD-2801/molnupiravir was unknown. But at least that drug was more stable than remdesivir and could be delivered with pills, though it appeared that, to be effective, the drug had to be delivered early in the illness.

Ridgeback took its promising drug to one of the largest multinational pharmaceutical companies in the world, Merck. During 2020, Merck withdrew the drug from the slow and regimented U.S. government-managed trials.

In the more detached way the United States handled drug development, Merck had the option of putting up the money to prepare its own clinical trials, taking on the investment risks. Without government help, Merck might need more time to do the work on its own but with more flexibility to line up with how Merck strategized about its own production timetable and the marketplace. Molnupiravir finally received an EUA (emergency use authorization) and became widely available to patients only in December 2021. That was two years after the pandemic began.

THE STRUGGLES OVER DRUG APPROVALS

Before any of these results from trials became known, the process for evaluating drugs had already become politically charged. The opening gun was the battle over whether Covid could be cured by an off-label use of hydroxychloroquine, an antimalarial repurposed to deal with some autoimmune disorders. TV hosts like Laura Ingraham praised it on Fox News. President Trump rushed to endorse it on television. The cry for hydroxychloroquine was itself a sign of the panic about Covid that was sweeping much of the country during the third week of March.

The government had not yet been able to rapidly organize high-quality trials of hydroxychloroquine. The president pressured his new FDA chief, Hahn, to approve the drug immediately and, if Hahn did not comply, the president urged HHS secretary Azar to look into ways to do the approval himself. Navarro started bombarding everyone with memos demanding immediate and massive reliance on hydroxychloroquine. In HHS, Giroir joined the push and Kadlec began pushing to buy stocks of the drugs.

Kadlec's subordinate, Bright, resisted, citing both safety concerns and unproven efficacy. The issue became a flashpoint of disagreement between the two men that included leaks by Bright to the press and soon led to Bright's departure from government. NIH leaders, including Fauci, also would not go along. Trump's former FDA leader, Scott Gottlieb, also tried to fight the panic.

The FDA quickly gave in. Woodcock, the center director, and Hahn both agreed to issue an EUA for use of the drug against Covid. The decision was not harmless; aside from some safety concerns, the new demand for the drug made it scarce for those who needed it for those other conditions. FDA career staff might have believed that an EUA designation would at least allow the government to start buying emergency supplies that could ease these shortages.

The publicity about the drug was so massive it became hard to organize scientifically valid clinical trials. Meanwhile, clinical evidence began accumulating. That evidence indicated that hydroxychloroquine was probably ineffective. The British study that demonstrated the value of dexamethasone for critically ill patients also showed that hydroxychloroquine did not seem to work. The WHO's trials confirmed that conclusion.

The FDA had granted an EUA for hydroxychloroquine on March 28. The EUA was revoked on June 15. The damage to the FDA's reputation was not so easily undone.[5]

During the summer of 2020 there was another bubble of enthusiasm, not grounded in prior experience, for using blood plasma from recovering patients ("convalescent plasma") as a treatment. Evidence on it ran back and forth, with many doctors believing that the treatment might help, but only if a patient received it before getting too sick. More-over, transfusing plasma from one patient to another can introduce complications and risk. Transfused plasma must also be screened for other diseases.

As the first wave of Covid moved across America during the summer, with health experts rightly predicting another wave in the colder months, President Trump and others again set up a cry, this time for approval of convalescent plasma. The NIH again would not go along. Yet, again, the pressure weighed on the FDA.

In September 2020 the relevant FDA center director, Peter Marks (who had played such a notable role in spurring the vaccine push), issued an emergency use authorization for convalescent plasma. Again, Hahn went along, and botched the public explanation of the reasons for his approval. This treatment also turned out to be ineffective in practice.[6]

This experience was, by all accounts, a difficult one for Hahn, who resolved that he and his agency would not be pushed around again. Pressure returned soon, as the Trump administration's supporters began raising the issue of a fast approval for the new vaccines making their way through tri-als, so the vaccines would be available in October (before the presidential election). Marks and Hahn refused to shortcut the process.

The consequences of these episodes were significant. The appearance of clashing evaluations of drug effectiveness from leaders opened the door for everyone (including a great many doctors, whatever their specialty) to form their own opinion. The cacophony only confused and hindered the vital process, necessary in any war, of picking the best weap-ons for the fight.

During the Biden administration, there were renewed arguments over the proper usage of booster vaccines. In August 2021, Woodcock, now the acting director of the FDA, agreed that Americans should start receiving boosters. Resenting yet another bout of political interference in their scientific decisions, the two leading officials in the vaccines office of the center headed by Marks resigned. They were not against boosters in principle, but they felt such shots were not yet needed for most vaccinated people and should, at that time, be reserved for high-risk populations or those, including people around the world, who were still unvaccinated.[7]

These episodes show the value of setting up a sound process for determining which weapons work best, including emergency trial setups, and then sticking by that process. Sometimes there are judgment calls to make and accountable officials must make them. But those should be people who have heard, understood, and evaluated the scientific and clinical arguments. The government process did not unduly delay the approval of good treatments. The few helpful treatments were more likely revealed by the process, as with dexamethasone in serious cases. It is not clear that any of the political interventions had any positive impact on public health.

THE BIOPHARMA INDUSTRIAL COMPLEX:
A BRIEF INTRODUCTION

The economics of the biopharmaceutical industrial complex involve huge up-front costs in development, manufacturing, and clinical trials. These later stages cost hundreds of millions of dollars. So firms wait for good evidence of a possible market that can repay those costs and make a profit.

Once the product is developed and approved, the marginal cost of making more of it might be small, but companies still run their numbers according to cost and profit. They try to get the best possible margins on their product prices, even if the marginal cost of making more is low, in order to pile up profits both to reward executives and investors and to pay for the costly research and development on new products that often don't pay off.

Headline companies, with names like Pfizer or Merck, are often lead partners or prime contractors. They might have a "discovery partner," a smaller firm that did the research and development to prepare a product and display its potential.

The big firms usually manage complex chains of companies, in various countries, that conduct their trials for them, supply heavyweight capital equipment like bioreactors, make materials like filters or pharmaceutical ingredients like adjuvants and lipids, or handle the jobs of doing the "fill and finish"—putting drugs or vaccines into vials and then packaging them for distribution.

To a health security executive, the challenge of managing the biopharma industrial complex might seem similar, at least in some ways, to the challenge of managing the defense-industrial complex that produces missiles, aircraft, tanks, or ships. In both areas—the biopharma industrial complex and the defense-industrial complex—much of the security business is based on advance government procurement of weapons. Such weapons are very difficult and costly to develop. They have complicated supply chains, ecosystems of contractors and suppliers. There is some regular demand for the products of these firms. But many weapons are bought in the hope that they will never be used in combat. So too with many drugs or vaccines or other specialized health security supplies.

The biopharma problem is harder than the defense-industrial problem. It is harder to predict the effectiveness of drugs and vaccines. Drugs have third-party regulators, like the FDA. Military equipment does not. Also, the government often buys military equipment with long-term contracts in which the product development is financed. Not so with drugs and vaccines.

In both areas, efforts do not turn out well if the firms build up manufacturing capabilities and then do not use them. The production lines and the skilled staff who operate them must at least be kept productive doing something useful, if those lines and staff are expected to perform at a high level in a crisis, perhaps spinning off new or expanded production lines.

The economics for drugs—for medicines—in a pandemic can sometimes factor in a large eventual demand. Once a lot of people get sick, there are a great many people, and governments, willing to pay for drugs that help them. Once that demand is there, companies will invest in developing the drugs. They will run production lines large enough to meet the demand. Yet again, though, the problem is harder than it seems: if demand is only perceived as a short-term spike, companies are less likely to invest. They might also worry that a cure-all vaccine may curb the disease and eliminate their market.

But all these calculations about possible market demand happen after the fact, after the demand has materialized. In a pandemic, that is too late. With a deadly infectious disease, people, and governments, usually want drugs fast, and in enormous quantities. Also, if the disease happens to disproportionately afflict people who cannot pay, governments or foundations may try to offset that market failure by stepping in to invest in development and production.

What we have said so far applies to drugs and vaccines. But the business model for making vaccines is different and harder than the business model for making drugs. Sick people are eager to buy drugs they think will help. Vaccines are preventive. The consumers aren't sick yet. Because they aren't sick, healthy people worry more about adverse effects from vaccines than sick people do about the side effects of drugs that make them well. Governments therefore try to make vaccines cheap or free. That means that governments provide more of the demand for vaccine products at every stage of the process.

HOW TO BUILD A BUSINESS BASE FOR A BIO EMERGENCY

Governments usually do not think of health as a security issue. They do not think about the task of producing medical countermeasures for a biowar in the way they have become accustomed to thinking about the task of producing very high-end military products. But the task of producing medical defenses can sometimes be even harder than traditional defense procurement.

Many citizens are accustomed to the idea that a defense industrial base that builds advanced weapons has many large companies and is very difficult to manage. Consider, then, the commercial partnerships and the capabilities that may be required to defend a country against biological threats, such as pandemics or a deliberate biological attack.

The United States, since 2002, is one of the few countries in the world that has even tried to orchestrate this kind of enormous innovation in the public interest. It is quite a task, one that now many other countries are also trying to take on.

The quest often begins with a small grant to an academic research center. Perhaps that center has a promising lead. The animal and human trials required to prove a concept come with a steep jump in the cost and risk of development. Often, the initial development is done by a small, inexperienced company that can attract government support and, ideally, venture capital.

If a treatment appears promising and there is a likely market for it, perhaps one of the big companies may step in. It can help produce the product, manage the extremely difficult and expensive animal and human clinical trials, and deal with all the regulators and other government issues.

Then come the problems of manufacturing. This involves very high-quality chemical or biological engineering on a large scale that must meet regulatory standards of "good manufacturing," able to avoid contamination. The supply chains for pharmaceutical products are complicated and extended, sometimes with hundreds of components.

It is a high-stakes business that tries to make huge profits on a few winners to offset the losses from the more common dead ends. Scientific, technical, financial, and regulatory failures litter the path to market. The mRNA technology that has been developed for vaccines offers the possibility of smaller-scale and faster manufacturing processes.

As we explained, the large companies that choose to navigate this path are only interested in products that have very large, promising markets. They are rarely interested in developing countermeasures for an emerging disease, or to counter some hypothetical biological weapon, where the future markets for some products are uncertain.

They must also ask themselves: If we develop this product, how will we prove that it works in order to get regulatory approval in advance of the need, that is, before there are widespread, or any, human cases of the disease?

Before the Covid war, only a small number of large pharmaceutical companies had assembled the needed production capabilities and supply networks. Big pharmaceutical companies were cautious about making huge investments in medicines or vaccines for emerging diseases. They knew that government interest in such threats cycles between panic and neglect. Yes, there would be panicked interest during the crisis. Then the panic would subside. The money would dry up. Companies risk losing their investments. It had happened before, with Ebola and other diseases.

When the government wants to invest in a defense capability, it may have to make a long-term commitment. For instance, HIMARS missiles have recently been in the news as crucial supplies for Ukraine's armed forces trying to throw back the Russian invaders. These missiles were first developed when the U.S. Army gave Lockheed Martin a $23 million contract to build four prototypes, back in 1996. More contracts supported development and testing. Initial production did not begin until 2003. The missiles are currently made at an industrial park in southern Arkansas run by Lockheed Martin, the fruit of this quarter-century commitment. The major pharmaceutical companies do not receive such commitments to produce health security products for which there is not yet a large demand. (And, as we will mention later, even HIMARS did not get the multi-year contract to be sure there would be enough of the missiles in a crisis.)

To illustrate some of the problems in waiting for a crisis to develop large business partnerships, it helps to go back to an earlier topic, the challenge of producing enough tests. South Korea had shown the way early in the Covid war, as it went straight into a public-private partnership to produce adequate numbers of tests. That approach seems very business friendly. It reflects a South Korean pattern of close government relationships with Korea's business champions. That has real risks. It has predictably embroiled its politicians in cases of favoritism and corruption.[8]

The initial American instinct is to be more detached from the firms. That might seem wiser. Yet that detachment can backfire. The American approach not only weakens the government's position when dealing with business; it increases reliance on only a few company options in an emergency. A more proactive health security strategy would identify the public needs and build relationships with a family of possible partners and suppliers.

In chapter 4, "Containment Fails; Mobilization Lags," and chapter 5, "Federal Crisis Management Collapses; Operation Warp Speed Begins," we described the more passive approach to producing tests in America, one that initially relied on government design and manufacture of Covid diagnostic tests and also tightly regulated initial production of both PCR and rapid antigen tests. That approach, which was nominally so detached from industry, ended up putting the big test production companies in a very strong position when the emergency hit.

The big testing production companies managed the approvals process on their own, and largely on their own terms. They produced tests with proprietary supply chains and proprietary components that could not be interchanged with tests made by their rivals. An Abbott swab might not work with a Labcorp reagent. So the whole testing system in America was cut up into proprietary stovepipes. Since almost all the little test developers at hospitals and labs could not produce and distribute at scale, they were not a competitive threat.

Therefore, in the American system, hundreds of tests got EUAs. Yet the market was utterly dominated by two or three big producers who made huge profits. In the South Korean system, only about twenty producers got the permits and all the business, but the marketplace was actually much more competitive and responsive to public needs.

The major public-private R&D entity to develop life-saving drugs for a bio emergency was BARDA. However, BARDA did not have the manufacturing capabilities to respond at scale in a crisis.[9]

Before the pandemic, Kadlec wanted to assess BARDA's readiness for a major emergency. He asked the MITRE Corporation, which operates six federally funded research and development corporations (or FFRDCs), to study BARDA and the whole medical countermeasures enterprise. After consulting with scores of executives outside of the government, MITRE briefed Kadlec in July 2019 and completed the project in November, just as the Covid outbreak was probably beginning in China. Their conclusion: the nation's medical countermeasures mission was at risk. It was unlikely to be able to handle likely future biological threats.[10]

The basic problem, MITRE found, was that BARDA did not build long-term partnerships to be sure the country would have an industrial base to produce at the speed and scale required in a crisis, with viable companies and supporting supply chains. It did not have the budget or the contracting authorities to make sustained commitments, even if it wanted to.

Firms needed long-term investments and predictable cash flow. If a Big Pharma firm is going to make a multi-year investment, protected from the cycle of panic and neglect, then it needs a multi-year commitment of funding. There once was a program to offer just such multi-year support. It was called Project BioShield. Yet, when BioShield was reauthorized in 2014, Congress converted its funding structure into a single-year appropriation that was supposed to be large enough to tempt companies to make long-term commitments, but not well designed to really manage these grants as partnerships.

Here is the big takeaway: investments in health security should be judged and organized on a national security standard. They do not necessarily contribute to routine healthcare. Yet, since a pandemic kills thousands and costs billions every day, the returns on investment, by almost any measure, might far exceed the returns from other national security spending.

The ASPR's funding for medical countermeasures was about one-fifth of what was being spent on missile defense. It was about one-eighth of what was being budgeted for cyber-security. Those numbers offer a rough approximation of how the U.S. government set its budget priorities for new threats. Those were the priorities before Covid.

When the Covid war began, the research part of the medical countermeasures enterprise moved very fast. It had two jobs: try to find a cure and try to find a vaccine. The first job was an immediate matter of life and death, since finding, developing, and distributing a vaccine was bound to take some time.

NO "WARP SPEED" FOR DRUGS

Why did the United States have such a sputtering record of success in trying to devise drugs to defeat COVID-19? The United States had not built the business base for a bio emergency. With drugs, it did not build that base during the war, either.

The prewar medical countermeasures enterprise had not built, or incentivized, the biopharma industrial base to enable rapid fielding of drugs in a large emergency. Even if potential drugs were being identified, the U.S. system did not bring in the clinical and operational partners, the physicians in the field, needed to help plan and guide how to deploy vital drugs at scale. Private companies alone could not prepare for emergency deployment of their products.

The two most promising treatment approaches to emerge by the autumn of 2020 were monoclonal antibodies and protease inhibitors. Very specific monoclonals replicated the proteins made by the immune cells that evolved to attack a particular virus.

This form of treatment can have a relatively short timeline for value. Certain monoclonals can become obsolete as the particular virus it was designed to beat evolves into new variants. Other monoclonal antibodies seem to retain broader effect against multiple variants. However, by the summer of 2022, only one FDA-authorized monoclonal therapy remained active against the latest variants (called BA.4 and BA.5).

Back in October 2020, both Regeneron and Eli Lilly had put their monoclonal treatments into government clinical trials. The bigger company, Lilly, eventually withdrew from the government process to do its own trials. Its product went on the market in 2021, until virus variants made it obsolete. Lilly later produced another monoclonal that remained promising at least into 2022.

The other promising approach in autumn 2020 was to use protease inhibitors. These affect the enzymes that the viruses use to mature. Their use is therefore closely linked to testing: the drugs need to be started in the early stages of infection, preferably within five days of first symptoms.

Several companies tried to find the right combination for such a protease inhibitor. Building on a drug of this kind originally developed in the SARS epidemic of 2002–04, Pfizer devised a protease inhibitor formulation (combining nirmatrelvir and ritonavir) that displayed great success in trials during 2021. The drug was called Paxlovid. It was also stable and could be taken orally. It became available for general use at the end of 2021, two years into the pandemic.

Such protease inhibitors were not available when President Trump himself was infected by COVID-19 at the beginning of October 2020. President Trump did benefit from the NIH's knowledge of which drugs were being developed.[11]

From publicly available evidence, it seems that President Trump became seriously ill. He was in a demographic profile with a significant risk of death. As soon as he was hospitalized, he received the Regeneron monoclonal antibody treatment. Some circumstantial evidence suggests he might have received the Lilly monoclonal too.

Both of these drugs were still in clinical trials, not available to the general public. President Trump's doctors applied for and received FDA permission for use of an "Emergency Investigational New Drug." This is allowed if the doctor feels the experimental drug is urgently needed for a serious or life-threatening condition.

President Trump's Regeneron dosage appears to have been more than twice the amount being used in the Regeneron trials. President Trump also received remdesivir. His condition became serious enough to warrant giving him dexamethasone as well. He recovered enough so that he soon felt able to leave the hospital.

The "therapeutics" side of the fight against COVID-19 highlights the fact that government preparations were unable to make a decisive difference during the first years of struggle. Although prior governmental R&D efforts did accelerate the arrival of several coronavirus antiviral drugs and monoclonal antibodies, they did not quickly make a large impact on COVID-19.

A good example comes from the experience with Covid monoclonals in late 2020. The earliest monoclonals approved for emergency use by the FDA (from Lilly and Regeneron) showed amazing efficacy in clinical trials. As they became more widely available, they were often used poorly and ineffectively. Healthcare providers did not use them on the patients who could benefit the most.

To have maximum impact, these monoclonals—for confirmed Covid patients—used a thirty-minute infusion that had to occur within the first days of illness to have maximum impact. The U.S. healthcare system was not set up to routinely conduct widespread diagnostic testing or provide large-scale outpatient IV infusions. In other words, the deployment of the drugs needed a targeted implementation plan to go with it. In November 2020, ASPR partnered with a few sites to create pilot programs for use of monoclonals. That helped, but it was too little, too late.

The monoclonals story illustrates that, in a war, it is not enough to evaluate and buy the weapons. People have to be prepared to use them effectively, in the right setting, or all that hardware might prove worthless.

In chapter 7, on the healthcare system, we discussed how important it was to learn and distribute guidance as doctors learned what clinical practices worked best. We suggested ways to improve that process. There is a similar issue with drug treatments. In the Covid war, the messaging—to the general public and to medical professionals—did not effectively communicate who should get what kinds of treatment, and why.

That weak messaging then had to fight against the deluge of misinformation about alternative therapies like hydroxychloroquine or ivermectin, which also turned out to be ineffective. The result was that even when some good treatments were abundant, which was the case by the spring of 2022, only a minority of the patients who qualified for and would have benefited from an anti-Covid drug actually received one.[12]

The U.S. government's Operation Warp Speed, which kicked off in the spring of 2020, did try to identify and accelerate effective drugs. It did this partly by sponsoring large-scale simultaneous trials of every promising candidate.

But, to retain control of the trials, the big multinationals did not buy into that process for the candidates that they decided to back. The major players, like Merck and Pfizer, set their own timeline, using their own judgment, for development of effective treatments. If the companies succeeded, what was left was for governments to negotiate with them about the scale of production and the price.

When the breakthrough finally occurred in 2021 with drugs like Paxlovid, the United States followed a peacetime approach. It did not adopt the Warp Speed approach. It did not make an advance market commitment to buy Pfizer's Paxlovid at a large scale until after Phase 3 trials had begun in the late autumn of 2021.

By that time, Pfizer had such decisive results—90 percent effectiveness—in its Phase 3 trial (in a high-risk group) that Pfizer and government overseers agreed that the trial should be stopped so the drug could be made available right away. Only at the point of Phase 3 success, at the beginning of November 2021, did the United States then commit to buy about 10 million courses of the drug, to be produced during 2022, at a cost of $5.3 billion.[13]

Therefore, only a tiny fraction of the courses was available when the Omicron wave of infections hit the United States and the rest of the world during the first half of 2022. On top of that, there was the earlier problem, shown with the monoclonals, that there were no national plans to guide and implement mass use of the treatment.

Physicians were surprisingly reluctant to prescribe Paxlovid, perhaps because its low and manageable risks were poorly understood. It is impossible to quantify how many more lives might have been saved if Paxlovid had been readily available early in 2022, with practical guidelines for its use, but the number would probably be substantial.

In a wartime approach, the U.S. government could have committed to the same scale of procurement months earlier, to be ready in the winter of 2021–22, or it could have decided to spend the money for an even larger procurement. Possible guidelines for wide use would have been readied. Pills might have been stockpiled and then not used, if the later trials were disappointing.

These are large multibillion-dollar bets. But they are the scale of the bets placed for vaccines in Operation Warp Speed.

We do not know why the U.S. government held off on a Warp Speed approach with Paxlovid and other drugs earlier in 2021. The funding commitments would have been very large, and Warp Speed had no regular funding. Most of its original funding had been transferred from another program.

In the spring and summer of 2021, both on the scale of investments in tests and its scale of investments in drugs, it seems as if the Biden administration's crisis managers thought the Covid war was waning, and then were caught off guard by the third (Delta) and fourth (Omicron) waves. The Biden administration's response on both testing and drugs was then very impressive during late 2021 and early 2022.

In wartime, governments place such procurement bets all the time. In the Covid war, governments should have placed such bets across a desired portfolio of capabilities (various kinds of vaccine platforms, various kinds of therapies, various kinds of diagnostics), accepting that some of the bets would not pay out. As we will show, Operation Warp Speed did this on a relatively small scale for vaccines.

If the United States made these big commitments, it could also have more leverage in writing contracts. It might, for example, have asked Pfizer to be willing to license manufacturing of Paxlovid as much as possible around the world. Based on its subsequent performance, Pfizer might have been willing to do this. Although vaccines have captured the world's attention, much of the world (and the United States) will not get vaccinated. Medicines still have their place.

UNDERSTANDING THE SUCCESS WITH VACCINES—AND OPERATION WARP SPEED

The vaccines success and Operation Warp Speed is more celebrated than understood. It does deserve close attention. The government role in this case was much more important and the policy design for government support was effective. But only up to a point.

The basic design of a vaccine engineered to target a coronavirus was built on years of direct and indirect public support. Within twenty-four hours of obtaining the gene sequence for COVID-19, a scientist at the NIH, Barney Graham, and a former colleague, then at the University of Texas, Jason McLellan, got right to work. They joined with colleagues in their labs, such as Nianshuang Wang (a Chinese citizen working in McLellan's lab), Daniel Wrapp, and Kizzmekia Corbett. They developed a plausible vaccine design by the end of January 2020. They could then work to test what they had done with government-sponsored coronavirus labs like those led by Baric at North Carolina and Denison at Vanderbilt.

The NIH quickly publicized and shared its breakthrough. The most novel technology to deliver such an engineered vaccine used messenger RNA (mRNA). This vaccine does not use a weakened or inactive form of the virus in order to trigger immune responses. It instead prompts cells to create a protein to produce the immune response.

This mRNA technology had been worked on for years by several scientists, mainly based in the United States but also in Europe. One company was based in Germany, BioNTech. It was headed by Uğur Şahin and Özlem Türeci, and it used the mRNA technology developed by the Hungarian-trained scientist Katalin Karikó and her American colleague, Drew Weissman. Karikó was working for BioNTech in Germany.

Another company, Moderna, had its own version of mRNA, developed by the American Derrick Rossi and modified by an Israeli-trained scientist, Tal Zaks, and his colleagues. The NIH, BARDA, and DARPA had spent years betting on and supporting Moderna as a test case of how to accelerate vaccine development.

There were two other approaches to a Covid vaccine. A viral vector vaccine would use a more benign virus, like an adenovirus, to convey instructions to cells that prompt the immune response. This kind of vaccine had been used before. A protein subunit vaccine uses parts of proteins in the Covid virus with an ingredient, called an adjuvant, that stimulates the immune system to respond to such proteins in the future. A protein subunit vaccine had been used successfully to counter hepatitis B. At the beginning of 2020, no one had ever successfully developed, manufactured, and used mRNA vaccines.

Each vaccine approach had risks of failure somewhere along the way. The regulators, like the FDA, did not have a deep base of knowledge and experience with any of them. Logically, a really ambitious vaccine program therefore had to invest in a portfolio of candidates, to hedge against the risk that some of them might falter.

Earlier in the book we noted how a number of people saw the chance to organize a massive vaccine project with this portfolio concept. Some of them used the analogy to the Army's Manhattan Project during the Second World War, the huge effort to build an atomic bomb as quickly as possible. In that story, a few scientists played a key role. They had to convince the people who ran the war effort that such a project was worth a colossally large bet.

In 1942 those top scientists, the validators who bridged the worlds of science and big policy choices to coach leaders on where to place their bets, were Vannevar Bush and James

Conant. In 2020, in the Covid war, Francis Collins and Anthony Fauci played the Bush-Conant role. Early work by their already established private partner, Moderna, helped Collins and Fauci see and make the scientific case.

At the same time, the BioNTech group in Germany also realized what might be possible, just as the Moderna group did. The BioNTech group reached out to Pfizer.

WARP SPEED IN ACTION

When it was organized by the U.S. Army, the Manhattan Project had paired a military commander of the project, General Leslie Groves, with a scientific leader of the project work, J. Robert Oppenheimer. When Operation Warp Speed was organized by Azar, working with Jared Kushner at the White House, they set up a similar operation.

In the Covid war the Groves role was played by General Gustave Perna. The Oppenheimer role was played by Moncef Slaoui (a former Big Pharma executive born in Morocco). President Trump and Kushner delegated the vital management tasks to Slaoui and Perna. The Defense Department took on much of the heavy administrative and operational burden of handling the contracting—the process of buying and building—as well as the process of deploying these new weapons.

Perna and Slaoui turned out to be highly capable leaders. They had a great deal of autonomy to run the project, with weekly updates to a board chaired by Kushner. The other key members of the Warp Speed leadership team were from

HHS (including one from the FDA and Collins at NIH), the Department of Defense, and two private sector experts in vaccine development and manufacturing.

The full policy design took form. It included a plan for investment in a portfolio of vaccines, hedging by betting strategically on a select set of candidates.

The U.S. government's relationship with Moderna illustrated just the kind of proactive public-private partnership that the MITRE study had proposed. In 2020 Moderna was being led by a French chief executive who kept the company afloat through thick and thin, mostly thin. The mRNA platform was promising but its potential had needed parallel work in an essential component: lipid nanoparticles to protect the mRNA and turn it into injectable doses. It was a Department of Defense component, the Defense Advanced Research Projects Agency (DARPA) that helped connect Moderna to a lipids company with that capability.

Other scientists used different vaccine designs and delivery systems. A group in the United Kingdom, centered at Oxford, was using adenoviruses to try the viral vector approach and deliver enough pieces of the coronavirus into the system to stimulate immunity. Also using adenoviruses was a group working with the Janssen division of the giant firm Johnson & Johnson.

The protein subunit approach, to create and inject entire proteins, a portion of the virus, to trigger the antibody reactions was also being tried. A small American company, Novavax, was trying to make that work.

At the beginning of 2020, none of the "discovery partners"—BioNTech, Moderna, or Novavax—had much experience with producing successful vaccines. None could

PLATFORM TECHNOLOGIES	mRNA PLATFORM	REPLICATION-DEFECTIVE LIVE-VECTOR PLATFORM	RECOMBINANT-SUBUNIT-ADJUVANTED PROTEIN PLATFORM
	Lipid nanoparticle / SARS-CoV-2 spike RNA	Viral vector / SARS-CoV-2 spike gene	SARS-CoV-2 spike protein
VACCINE CANDIDATES	Moderna Pfizer-BioNTech	Oxford-AstraZeneca Janssen/Johnson & Johnson	Novavax Sanofi-GSK

A diagram showing the six COVID-19 vaccine candidates supported by Operation Warp Speed and the platform technology used by each. Adapted from U.S. Government Accountability Office, "Operation Warp Speed: Accelerated COVID-19 Vaccine Development Status and Efforts to Address Manufacturing Challenges," GAO-21-319 (February 2021).

produce vaccines on an industrial scale. They had to get a Big Pharma partner to do that or else build up such an enormous capacity overnight.

The net result, guided by Slaoui, was that the U.S. government invested in three vaccine platforms with two producers on each. They were mRNA (Moderna, Pfizer-BioNTech); adenovirus viral vector (Oxford-AstraZeneca and Janssen/Johnson & Johnson); and protein subunit (Novavax and Sanofi-GSK).

Neither Moderna nor Novavax had big industrial partners to handle the manufacturing. In both cases, the government tried to help solve the problem, with more success for Moderna.

Merck tried to produce a vaccine using a viral vector platform and an adaptation of a measles vaccine it had developed with the Pasteur Institute. Those efforts were unsuccessful. Merck dropped out of the Warp Speed program early in 2021.

The U.S. officials argued about whether to go with this portfolio approach or concentrate on the protein subunit platform. Slaoui insisted on investing across the full portfolio. He won the argument. The first really big advance purchase commitment (on May 21, 2020) went to Oxford-AstraZeneca.

The Warp Speed policy design included planning to manage the trials. It included still more careful planning, using the authorities of the Defense Production Act, to secure the supply chains for everyone, especially some of the smaller companies that did not have Big Pharma's established network and clout.

The policy design also included planning for distribution to the states and harnessing private sector networks, like the big drugstore chains, to accomplish this. The officials working on Warp Speed argued about whether they should rely on state and local public health departments to distribute and administer the vaccines or rely more on a complex set of public-private partnerships with the big drugstore companies. General Perna chose the public-private approach, including work with the major pharmacy chains. This was the design that Anita Patel, at CDC, did so much to help develop.

The Pfizer-BioNTech partnership, however, tried to stay clear from the Operation Warp Speed program. Pfizer declined up-front support. Mango, in his memoir of his work with Operation Warp Speed, said that "of all the companies in which we invested, Pfizer was both the least transparent and least collaborative."[14]

Pfizer has deep pockets, an executive team from around the world, and extensive global partnerships, allowing it to rely more on its own money and capabilities. Its executives had plenty of experience in working with the U.S. government on pandemic preparedness, much of it unhappy. They made their own strategic decisions and ran their own trials, while of course keeping an eye on the others. Pfizer, like some other companies, was also negotiating purchase commitments with other governments.

Therefore, the Covid war saw a kind of natural experiment in how to develop and produce the mRNA vaccine. For Moderna, Operation Warp Speed was the essential partner. But Pfizer, on the other hand, could argue that its development timeline would have unfolded in about the same way, whether or not the Americans had created an Operation Warp Speed—and Pfizer delivered two weeks faster than Moderna.

Pfizer did encounter manufacturing and supply chain problems in the last months of 2020. It found that its possible U.S. suppliers had already been claimed by other Warp Speed producers who could push all rivals aside with the powers they had working with the Defense Production Act. To clear those bottlenecks, Pfizer then went through the process and made the disclosures required to get Warp Speed's authorities too. During 2021, Pfizer did eventually master its own path to ramp up production free of U.S. government constraints.

The Covid war has been immensely profitable for Moderna and Pfizer. For example, Pfizer's revenue in 2021 was more than $80 billion, doubling its 2020 revenue. Its mRNA vaccine formulations have majority market share in the

United States and Europe, and Paxlovid is the best early stage Covid drug. In 2022 the Covid vaccines and drugs alone are expected to bring in more than $50 billion in revenue, worldwide. Pfizer has gained growing influence over the nature and timing of future Covid vaccines.[15]

Pfizer determined what the United States could buy out of its total planned global production. Pfizer determined who it would sell the vaccine to, and in what order—and deftly worked around the Defense Production Act when that constricted its freedom.

Constant experiments in government-funded labs, including a lab that one of us helped lead, showed the gradual loss of vaccine effectiveness against new variants. Companies like Pfizer could balance cost and public health risk in deciding when to invest in updating their existing and very successful vaccines.

It was also up to governments to join those conversations and help make those judgments. If the decisions were simply left to corporate leaders, public interests might align with private interests, or they might not.

In sum, Operation Warp Speed was the best marriage of policy design and operational implementation of the Covid war. Its success was remarkable and fortunate. "Lucky" would not be too strong a word. The world was lucky that the first non-flu pandemic since HIV-AIDS was a coronavirus, a virus family for which the R&D community was relatively well prepared. The mRNA vaccine platform had never before been used successfully to counter a disease. It worked. If the mRNA platform had not worked as well as it did, there were others, and still are, but with different timelines and different levels of effectiveness.

PREPARING FOR THE FUTURE

In 2016, President Obama's science advisers urged him to build up a powerful set of medical weapons to counter a possible pandemic or bioattack. Their goal was to get to a level of pandemic readiness such that "not more than 6 months will be required to design, develop, manufacture, clinically test, and license vaccines and antibodies against many types of pathogens." In the United States and around the world, the deadliest phase of the pandemic began in the autumn of 2020, well over six months after the outbreak had begun.[16]

That 2016 vision was not a pipe dream. We believe it is possible to build a portfolio of vaccine, therapeutic, and diagnostic weapons readied for quick action in the next public health crisis. For instance, in developing vaccines, experts recognized years ago that the mRNA vaccine platform might be so flexible, and so much easier to manufacture at scale, that it could enable astonishing new capabilities. That is why NIH leaders and BARDA, with help from Defense Department research agencies, were keeping companies like Moderna afloat. There was no big business proposition for a large infectious disease vaccine development effort. BioNTech had stayed afloat by attracting investment in the possibility of an application against cancer.

To attract high-performing private sector partners and build such a portfolio of medical countermeasures, the executive leaders of the national biological security effort will need to tailor the right partnerships. The idea of such partnerships might evoke an image of a government industrial policy for the biopharma sector. In this case the goal is not to pick winners and losers. The job is to connect and coordinate needed partners, in advance, even if they may end up competing with each other, as happened in Operation Warp Speed.

Different firms or different science projects need different incentive structures and business models, using tools such as grants, prizes, development support, or advance purchase commitments. Contracts can contain clauses to ensure speed, scale, and access in emergencies.

Rather than just building up a passive stockpile, leaders will need to learn how to (and who can) scale up fast in a crisis. Using hypothetical or actual pathogens, they will continuously need to exercise teams doing research, development, and manufacturing on demand.

The U.S. government and global partners could set national plans each year, using the scouting reports already being generated by the global Coalition for Epidemic Preparedness Innovation (CEPI) to identify the manufacturing teams, procedures, and platforms that can generate new vaccines within a hundred days.

Operation Warp Speed provided a model of how to combine exceptional leadership and an integrated command structure for rapid action. This program did not bypass existing government. It used it. It combined key figures at HHS with the right people from the Pentagon and talents from the private sector. It combined government with a wide set of private sector partners to drive every part of the medical countermeasures process. Deep knowledge from long-term basic research was integrated with practical operations.

Warp Speed's scientific leader, Slaoui, was given the budget, autonomy, and authority required to work across agencies to design the portfolio of desired investments. He and his aides could make rapid go or no-go decisions on the basis of new and changing information from private sector developers and government agencies.

After Slaoui left in 2021, the program lost some of this autonomy and agility to make midcourse corrections. Slow to respond to variants of concern, Pfizer and Moderna eventually issued bivalent boosters on their own terms, but only after advocating four rounds of vaccines targeting the original strain. Pfizer and Moderna, quite understandably, did not want to hastily (from their point of view) put aside the existing demand for their products. Neither company committed to the more costly and risky program of developing a variant-proof vaccine or vaccines that block transmission, either of which would be a game changer.

The NIH and the FDA overcame this reluctance. The FDA, in particular, successfully pushed both Pfizer and Moderna toward deployment of a bivalent vaccine that would both renew old immunities and protect against some new variants.

A different way of buying medical countermeasures needs a different way of appropriating the money to buy them. Most of the money to fund Operation Warp Speed was not appropriated for it. In other words, there is no established pipeline of congressional appropriations to sustain a Warp Speed-type program in the present, or the future.[17]

How the U.S. government writes its contracts matters too. The Ukraine war has drawn intense attention to the remarkable performance of HIMARS missiles, but also to how few of them the Pentagon has on hand. Explaining the problem, a top Pentagon official, a man named Bill LaPlante, who, among other things, oversees the weapons-buying to save Ukraine, pointed out that "what really matters is contracts."[18]

The problem, LaPlante noted, was that "we don't do multi-year contracts [for these missiles]. We do multi-year contracts for ships. We do it for airplanes. We don't do it for these other [things]. We need to do it because that'll stabilize the supply chain."

LaPlante commented that multi-year contracts "send a signal to industry to say: They [in government] are in it for the long haul, and we can make the commitment." He added: "And so, what that means—this is a culture shift for us, as a country—we have to be comfortable as taxpayers funding production lines to produce things that the U.S. may never use. And that's something that we as a country have to struggle with."

What this Pentagon leader said about missiles made by Lockheed applies equally well to antiviral medicines made by Pfizer or a vaccine made by GSK or a diagnostic test designed by Abbott. This sort of approach to emergency readiness involves executive policy to do multi-year contracts.

Then Congress has to authorize money on such a multi-year basis. Another part of Congress has to appropriate money on the same multi-year basis. Multi-year contracts and appropriations offer more opportunities for rigidity and abuse. There are plenty of stories about wasted money and poor decisions in buying ships and aircraft. Those are hard problems. But the solution is not to quit buying ships and aircraft.

Restrictive funding statutes may seem arcane. But, as much as anything else in government, they are what limit the ability of the United States to prepare adequately for pandemics. We can imagine a system that would encourage Warp Speed approaches that cut across agency boundaries and congressional committee jurisdictions, that offer flexibility in the tools to use with industry and engage internationally with global partners.

Congressional committees jealously guard their power to authorize and appropriate funds. This is understandable.

Those who want to change the system might encourage Congress instead to use its powers of oversight. Private firms know perfectly well that even multi-year contracts do not exempt them from oversight of their performance. The balance of power within Congress may need to shift from appropriators to authorizers and overseers. The appropriations committees will still have plenty of work to do.

10

STRATEGY FOR A
GLOBAL WAR

THIS CHAPTER IS about the global war effort. Most of the containment or non-medical measures had to work at the national or local level. Yet the key medical countermeasures, above all vaccines, that were crucial to the health of the whole world were produced by only a few countries.

The quality of international cooperation in the Covid war has been disappointing. Some failings have been offset by the improvisation of private individuals, like the Chinese scientist Zhang Yongzhen who, without authorization, first shared the COVID-19 genome with the outside world. Sometimes the failings have been mitigated by the workings of private multinational partnerships or private nonprofits.[1]

On a large political scale, the key countries never adequately created an allied war effort against the virus. The World Health Organization's disappointing performance did not cause that failure. Constrained by choices of its member governments, the WHO reflected their failure.

One unique feature of the global vaccines effort is an exceptional role for nonprofit, non-governmental institutions.

Observers had long noticed that the market failed to provide what many people in the world might need to prepare for a health emergency, especially vaccines, and especially in poorer countries. At the end of the 1990s, the Bill & Melinda Gates Foundation organized a group of founding partners who would shoulder the burden of some of this biological defense procurement. They would make advance commitments to buy vaccines in order to encourage development and improve access for poor countries.

In 2000, that initiative became the Global Alliance for Vaccines and Immunization—now known as Gavi, the Vaccine Alliance. Its core partners, with the Gates Foundation, were the WHO, UNICEF, and the World Bank. Twenty years later, Gavi was providing vaccinations for almost half of the world's children.[2]

Gavi built up routine public health. But the Ebola outbreak of 2014–15 in West Africa, which killed thousands of people, spotlighted the need for biological defense procurement. A completely effective vaccine for Ebola had been under development for a decade but was not ready when the crisis hit.

In the United States after 9/11, Congress and the Bush 43 administration had created a vehicle for this kind of anti-outbreak biological defense procurement; that was the agency with the acronym BARDA (Biomedical Advanced Research and Development Authority), established in 2006, which we have discussed before. Nonprofit foundations interested in health security, like the Bill & Melinda Gates Foundation and the Wellcome Trust, saw how markets failed to provide these critical countermeasures and they noticed the U.S. precedent in creating BARDA.

These foundations, along with Norway, India, and the World Economic Forum, created the unusual nonprofit we have mentioned before, the Coalition for Epidemic Preparedness Innovation (CEPI). Gavi was still the global nonprofit doing vaccine procurement, but it now had a global nonprofit R&D partner in CEPI to help prepare for outbreaks.

CEPI is headquartered in Oslo, with offices in London and Washington, DC. In addition to foundation support, CEPI pools resources for epidemic vaccine innovation from about thirty countries, including the United States. CEPI's job was, and is, to identify areas where vaccine investments can do the most good and to nurture the seedlings.

Led by a member of this group, Richard Hatchett, CEPI is one of the institutions that scored a strategic success in preparing for the Covid war. It had identified coronaviruses as a major potential threat. It spotted mRNA technology as potentially useful against coronaviruses and invested in that, too. These relatively modest investments turned out to make a difference in speeding along the development of vaccines. But CEPI was not designed to do rapid scale-up and manufacturing. That required industrial partnerships for production and distribution.

AMERICA ALONE, COVAX, EUROPEAN CHOICES, AND SURPRISING SUCCESS

As we recounted in chapter 5, right at the outset of the pandemic, in February and March 2020, Richard Danzig and his informal, influential network had pressed hard for a massive effort to make vaccines rapidly available to the world.

They had imagined bringing together major governments like the United States, India, China, and Japan. Danzig advocated for doing this through CEPI. He argued that a non-governmental organization had a much better chance of being able to operate at the required speed.

In his original April 2020 discussion with Kadlec about the program that became Operation Warp Speed, the FDA's Peter Marks had shared this global vision. He too thought that the United States might reach out to a group like CEPI as a platform for organizing a global coalition effort.

These insights were fundamental and powerful. The viral enemy was global. Neither the United States nor any other country could separate its health from the health of a world in which the virus could freely proliferate and mutate into more dangerous forms.

Not only would a global effort have been appropriate for a global war, with large practical payoffs, but it would also have set an extraordinary precedent for world politics. It would show how countries might organize to meet new threats. Such a coalition effort could also have had large practical payoffs.

In April 2020, as the Warp Speed idea made its way from Kadlec to Azar to Kushner and to President Trump, U.S. officials put aside the global vision. Operation Warp Speed was designed to put America's needs first.

Meanwhile, also in April, the network of people Danzig had helped gather—especially Farrar, Hatchett, Venkayya, and Dzau, joined by Seth Berkley, the CEO of Gavi—moved out quickly to create a global structure specifically for Covid work. With particular support from the governments of France and Singapore, they partnered with the WHO to

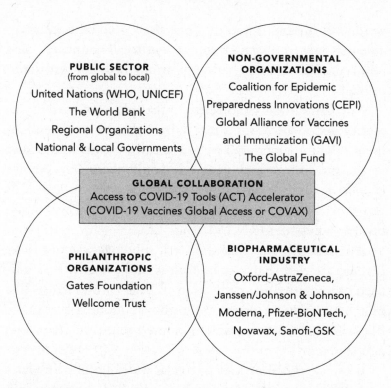

This diagram shows the sectors involved in global collaboration on the development and distribution of therapeutics and vaccines. Governments at all levels, non-governmental organizations, philanthropies, and the private biopharmaceutical industry all have important roles to play. During the Covid pandemic, emergency organizations like the Access to COVID-19 Tools (ACT) Accelerator were created to try to help coordinate these different sectors.

create the Access to COVID-19 Tools (ACT) Accelerator with a key vaccine pillar: an alliance for COVID-19 Vaccines Global Access, shortened as COVAX.

COVAX had some special features, different from Warp Speed or a typical national program. Its leaders imagined it

264 * LESSONS FROM THE COVID WAR

would buy billions of vaccine doses that could be made available not only to poorer countries, but to all countries based on need. COVAX also had some strong hedging features in mind.

As COVAX was established, in the spring and early summer of 2020, there was a real danger that vaccine development might not work out well. Typically, vaccine candidates at the preclinical trial stage have only about a 7 percent chance of success; even those that made it to clinical trials had only about a 20 percent chance. No one had ever developed a successful mRNA vaccine, yet.[3]

Another risk was that the work might take more time. Danzig showed that a six-month goal was realistic if pursued with wartime dedication. Other proponents, like Hatchett, thought twelve to eighteen months was more likely, though still others thought even that time frame was a pipe dream.

COVAX therefore had a broader portfolio of candidates than Warp Speed. COVAX eventually had contracts with eleven candidates and reserved rights to purchase from others. Thus, if there were problems in trials, COVAX would still be pooling risk and raising the odds that a collective investment would pay off. And, if production ramped up too slowly, COVAX could help distribute the fewer available vaccines to areas of greatest medical need, rich or poor.

By May 2020 there were then parallel structures: America's Operation Warp Speed and the global ACT Accelerator, which included COVAX. Warp Speed began picking its portfolio of vaccine candidates, led by science adviser Slaoui. COVAX began identifying its candidates, too, led by CEPI, headed by Hatchett. These lists overlapped with but were not identical to the Warp Speed list.

COVAX immediately fell behind because of funding. Warp Speed had ready money from America's federal government, which diverted money that had been appropriated to other programs. None of the COVAX funders, led by Gavi, were able or willing to draw down their cash reserves on a very large scale—billions of dollars—in the emergency. COVAX had to raise new money from governments and foundations. This took months.

Meanwhile, key European governments were not standing still. The British government decided to step out on its own, with a program analogous to Warp Speed, that was ably led and designed well.

The European Union held a pledging conference to raise money for an international Manhattan Project on vaccines and drugs. The goal was to get pledges of $8 billion. This effort slowed as the European Commission tried to reconcile the desires of twenty-seven national health authorities in organizing its collective procurement effort. Unlike the British, who were going their own way rather effectively, the EU did not use emergency procedures. It required that vaccines be fully certified by the European Medicines Agency. Within the EU, only Hungary adopted a mainly national approach to vaccine approval and procurement, turning to Russian and Chinese vaccines.[4]

Instantly tracking what the United States was doing (Warp Speed was announced in mid-May 2020) and what was happening with COVAX, and impatient with the European Commission's somewhat sluggish pace, about two weeks after the Warp Speed announcement, four European governments—France, Germany, the Netherlands, and Italy—announced that they would move ahead, working together to identify promising candidates and write contracts. The European Commission then followed their leads, starting to sign contracts by the end of August. These European decisions, following the U.S. example, made it clear that national, more self-interested, programs would lead the way, not the kind of collective global response embodied by COVAX.[5]

By the late summer of 2020, the first phases of clinical trials showed which vaccine candidates were showing promise. The lead national governments, then the European Commission, all zeroed in on them and signed their contracts. The United States, out front with the earliest advance market commitments, was at the head of the line. As it raised its money, COVAX fell in at the back of this initial queue. Meanwhile, China and Russia were producing their own products.

In many ways, this story turned out astonishingly well. Warp Speed's tighter portfolio of candidates turned out to include multiple winners. As its leaders might acknowledge, they were both lucky and good. Thanks in part to organizations like the NIH and CEPI, much good work had been done on coronaviruses before the crisis. The mRNA candidates were triumphant rookie successes for that technology. The timelines for product development and successful trials met the most optimistic predictions, taking about eleven months from the time developers got the genetic sequence of the virus to the first emergency authorization by a stringent regulator (Pfizer being authorized by Britain's regulator).

Private industry ramped up to produce vaccine doses on a scale that also triumphantly exceeded all predictions of what could be done. One reason was that mRNA vaccines were easier to manufacture. But the private organization of the multinational supply chains, often aided by national governments, still succeeded beyond most expectations.

In the pre-pandemic year, 2019, all vaccine production in the world totaled 5 billion doses. COVAX hoped that, by the end of 2021, the world might be able to produce 4 or 5 billion doses of the new Covid vaccines alone. That would have only been enough to provide adequate doses for about 30 percent of the global population, forcing difficult decisions about allocation. But, in fact, 11 billion doses of Covid vaccines were produced by the end of 2021. Covid vaccine production alone was thus more than twice as large as all vaccine production for all diseases in 2019.[6]

The national governments that led production of the vaccines prioritized vaccinating all of their people before vaccinating almost any people elsewhere, even those whose health was most vulnerable or whose work (like healthcare workers) left them most exposed. The concentration of vaccine manufacturing capability in four highly populated areas of the world—the United States, Europe, India, and China—made it certain that the needs of those areas would be served first.

There is still not a single Covid vaccine manufacturer in the Middle East. There is only one in sub-Saharan Africa. Analysts underestimated needs in poor countries, having little data about the impact of Covid in regions like Africa.

The national approach therefore threatened to devastate equitable access to vaccines. Yet the scale of production was so enormous that, by the end of 2021, the supply of vaccines saturated global demand. India contributed huge production and was part of global planning—a key partner in production of the Oxford-AstraZeneca vaccine.

China was also a huge producer, but on its own, with a more problematical vaccine design. China and Russia were going their own ways, pledging to produce doses for friendly nations ("vaccine diplomacy").

By 2022, supply was no longer the main obstacle to vaccine uptake anywhere in the world. COVAX was able to help. Backed with money raised by Gavi, COVAX ended up spending about as much on vaccines as Warp Speed did, but it raised and spent the funds over two years instead of in one. These were monumental achievements.

THE VALUE OF GLOBAL ACTION

We of course assume that, in an emergency, national governments will make huge purchases from necessary companies. They are likely to find that their companies, and the discovery partners and the supply chains, are usually not "one country" concerns. Those who try to keep it all in one country (like China) are more likely to develop inferior products.[7]

To cooperate on a large scale in an emergency, the preparations must be readied ahead of time. If major governments cooperate, they could develop global targets. They could then share the load of how to hit those targets. They could coordinate which supply chains they might commandeer and join in negotiating prices with the big firms.

In April 2020, U.S. officials could have met with key allied counterparts and offered to share the burden of the advance market commitments. They could have conferred about who would subsidize whom and worked on common principles in their contracts. They could have set joint procurement targets that had the world's eventual needs fully in view. The World Trade Organization's Secretariat had an infrastructure for such exchanges that had a good reputation for keeping company information secret.

Gavi and CEPI can be improved. But they were a pre-existing setup that could have been used to help organize and sustain a global coalition on a much larger scale in April and May 2020. There was, sadly, no chance that the Trump administration of 2020 could have led the organization of such a pathbreaking global coalition. Predictably, that U.S. government preferred to go it alone. President Trump in fact withdrew the United States from the World Health Organization, blaming it for supposed complicity in the "China virus."

The WHO and other international organizations struggled to organize the Access to COVID-19 Tools Accelerator (ACT-Accelerator) and most of its effort just went into vaccines, through COVAX. COVAX was a positive miracle of improvisation. Created in hectic times, it has organized the purchasing and delivery of nearly 2 billion vaccine doses around the world.[8]

In other words, amidst so much dismal hand wringing about problems with international organizations, these efforts actually suggest what is possible. A quickly improvised creation like COVAX was the principal reason a substantial fraction of people in low-income countries were vaccinated at all. Also, since the immunization programs in those countries were geared to children, it took another feat of international improvisation, helped by organizations like UNICEF, to help so many national governments also get Covid jabs to their older citizens most in need.

Yet these were triumphs of improvisation after the crisis had already begun. The key national leaders, starting with the United States, did not give programs like the ACT-Accelerator and COVAX a central place in their initial national plans. The result was that the ACT-Accelerator and COVAX effectively lost at least a year's worth of possible progress, fighting against vaccine hoarding, export restrictions, and problems with manufacturers.

A group of scholars led by Tom Bollyky and Jennifer Nuzzo pointed out that "these delays translate into millions of avoidable hospitalizations and deaths. They are mainly the result of inadequate global supplies of vaccine doses, and the challenges of planning, resourcing and implementing vast vaccination programs in countries with already strained health systems."[9]

Governments, including the United States and China, and foundations gave money to COVAX, which only then could make deals to buy a portfolio of vaccines and arrange to distribute them. COVAX has strained to get the funds it needs. Because Gavi and others were not able or willing to draw on their own pre-crisis cash reserves, COVAX also did not have the capacity to make advance market commitments. The wealthier national governments then tied up most of the initial supplies being produced through much of 2021.

Vaccine nationalism is understandable. The advantage of a global coalition of major vaccine or drug producers is not that the coalition leaders would ignore the needs of their own people. It is that they could form a plan, from the start, that would take the world into account.

Absent such planning, what tended to happen was that countries hoarded their own supplies until they were sure they would have a surplus, then they might offer them up to COVAX. But it takes time to set up vaccine education campaigns, distribution networks, cold chain storage facilities, and people ready to do the work.

"AMERICA FIRST" BACKFIRES

In the short run, the America First vaccine strategy seemed to pay off for Americans. The U.S. government dominated industrial production for its needs. In 2021, American citizens had better access to better vaccines than the citizens of any other country in the world.

Then the approach began to backfire. First, it backfired for American business. The Defense Production Act requirements actually discouraged production for non-Americans. Therefore, as they moved to serve the whole world, the main vaccine producers relied on businesses outside of America for those larger and longer-term global production plans.

U.S. vaccine production peaked right away, having made its U.S. deliveries. Soon, the vaccine production in the EU overtook the United States. Pfizer and Moderna moved production overseas to circumvent the America First provisions that were tied to the federal aid that had given those companies their first mover advantage. As Chad Bown pointed out: "European supply chains provided 160 percent more total doses than the United States." Even Pfizer-BioNTech and Moderna "each added much more production capacity to their supply chains in Europe than they did in the United States."[10]

India alone produced 40 percent more vaccines (mostly AstraZeneca) than did all the U.S. production in 2021 combined, though India kept much of its production to meet its own crisis. What happened was that, using the special powers of the Defense Production Act, the U.S. producers set up capacity to produce only for the U.S. government's orders. The U.S. government had only ordered for U.S. use. So, as they aimed at the whole global market, Pfizer and Moderna chose to partner with European producers to ramp up capacity to produce not only for Europe but for the world.[11]

Had the contracts in both the United States and Europe been designed differently and been better coordinated from the start, they could have leveraged public investment to ramp up capacity to produce on a global scale. U.S. producers would have been part of the game to make vaccines for the whole world, not just the United States, and they would have both made more money and also helped the world. There could have been far more vaccines available to organizations, like COVAX, that were eager to distribute them.

In July 2021 the Biden administration grasped the problem. It contracted for Pfizer to produce another 500 million doses for the rest of the world. But that contract still did not require Pfizer to ramp up production capacity, so the new U.S. order just took its place at the back of the queue.[12]

Having limited global opportunities for American business, the America First strategy then compromised U.S. leadership in the global Covid war.

From the start, the leading governments should have been coordinating their efforts for combating the next deadly virus. CEPI, created in 2016, has turned out to be a successful prototype for global sponsorship of proactive research and development.

Then, once at war, the U.S. government could have joined with allies, like the European Union's new Health Emergency Preparedness and Response Authority (created in September 2021) to drive global requirements for resilient portfolios of vaccines, therapeutics, and diagnostics. This coalition would then drive global coordination of national investments.

We expect that coalition participants, like the United States and the EU, would have set targets and timetables to prioritize vaccine deliveries for their own citizens. But, in this coalition approach, the plans would have fully taken global needs into account from the start, recognizing the common threat if the virus raged unchecked everywhere else in the world.

If COVAX had been fully funded and operational from the outset, it could have made large advance market commitments too. Knowing when supplies might arrive, COVAX and COVAX recipient countries would have been able to make delivery and education plans instead of trying to cope with unexpected, ad hoc donations.

The allies should have set evolving specifications for what they wanted in quantity and quality across portfolios for vaccines, drugs, and diagnostics. The allies should have begun coordinating their procurements and supply chain management. They should have begun setting targets for what would be needed on a global scale, not just for their own communities. Vaccine production encountered supply chain issues across the world that required countries to coordinate their subsidies, figuring out how to set prices or guaranteed purchases to ramp up availability of inputs like lipid nanoparticles or bioreactor bags.

THE POTENTIAL FOR U.S. LEADERSHIP OF A GLOBAL COALITION

Over the last hundred years, little of significance has happened in global health without U.S. leadership. The U.S. government did make large contributions to COVAX. But had the Biden administration stepped up to own the global Covid response as the Bush 43 administration did with HIV/ AIDS, a stronger coalition might have taken shape during 2021. That was the argument for proposals like the one in August 2021 from the Covid Collaborative, Duke University, and other partners for the Emergency Plan for Global COVID-19 Relief. What emerged instead, months later, was a modest global vaccination initiative from the U.S. Agency for International Development.

The Biden administration at least recognized the problem. It promptly rejoined the World Health Organization in 2021. It issued a flurry of public initiatives: a global Covid summit in 2021, another in 2022. It announced a U.S.-EU initiative to work on coordinating global manufacturing and supply chains, though this has not yet led to any substantive results.

The Biden administration also began reestablishing a reasonably orderly day-to-day crisis management effort led by its new coordinator, Jeff Zients. But the Biden administration did not develop an adequate, practical strategy to win the global Covid war. It did not develop a wartime coalition approach for the development, production, and delivery of medical countermeasures on a global scale.

The net result was that, by late 2022, the global production of vaccines was on the right scale but still not well coordinated to meet global needs. A global outlook goes back to the way leaders put together their portfolios for investment.

Both Warp Speed and COVAX made bets on the non-mRNA vaccines made by Johnson & Johnson, Oxford-AstraZeneca, and Novavax. Initially some bets turned out better than others. That was foreseeable; that is why the right approach was to invest across a broad portfolio. But, with a global perspective, speed to market is only one of the priorities. Other priorities would be usability in different parts of the world.

For instance, one of the mRNA vaccines, made by Pfizer-BioNTech, had a difficult cold chain storage challenge. Moderna's was only a little easier. But the Johnson & Johnson vaccine was much easier to transport and store. That would be a global factor.

Also, the protein subunit vaccine, Novavax, had production difficulties and therefore was not a high priority for the U.S. and European consumers. But Novavax still commanded interest from a global perspective because it was much easier to transport and store. It might have been prioritized for Asian or African markets where cold chain requirements posed such problems.

Or, to take another example, the U.S. FDA refused to endorse the Oxford-AstraZeneca vaccine because of concerns about blood clots. This decision was a close call from a purely U.S. point of view, given the alternatives available to

U.S. consumers. But this debatable decision had large effects on the uptake of this vaccine in parts of the world that could have used it, given that it was easier to transport and store.

Also, given the difficulties with vaccine uptake in much of the world, life-saving therapeutics should also have been a high priority from the start. We have already criticized the absence of a Warp Speed for therapeutics, such that they were not sufficiently available even in the United States. And, because resources were deferred from a global point of view as well, when Paxlovid cleared its clinical trials in late 2021, the rest of the world had to get in line behind the United States, which had already waited to buy the drug.

As in the Second World War, the Covid war relied on a few major powers to help the rest of the world. If the handful of biological superpowers were to see their responsibility appropriately, they would also see that the rest of the world would, eventually, be a vital part of what would be needed in the future—for biomedical intelligence, necessary supplies, and a global set of partners and talent. That sense of responsibility would pay dividends, tangible and intangible, over time. The returns on investment, even in narrow economic terms, would be very great.

The United States, the major European countries, and the major Asian powers have not yet joined forces effectively enough. Led by the charitable examples from Europe and the United States, they were eventually willing to donate what they could spare. But their original procurement and distribution plans were not designed with the world in mind. And, from the start, the Covid war has been a global war.

11

AMERICA THE COMPETENT?

I N AN EARLY book about the pandemic, with the uplifting title *Doom*, Niall Ferguson thoughtfully observed that "pandemics, like world wars and global financial crises, are history's great interruptions. . . . they are also moments of revelation." One reason the American response to the pandemic was discouraging was because, at least at times and to many, our governance was seemingly revealed to have been so incompetent. If citizens do not believe their government can handle the largest emergencies, the republic is in trouble.[1]

That revelation was particularly distressing because it was the latest stumble in a series of tragic stumbles, including the catastrophes in Iraq and Afghanistan. And this was the performance of a country that once justifiably regarded itself, and was regarded by many non-Americans, as being best in world in handling large emergencies. America had been the exemplar of can-do, practically minded, public accomplishment.

We have shown that, during the Covid war, a great many Americans actually did end up displaying that kind of will and know-how. One reason we wrote this book was to add that revelation, too: to notice these outstanding improvisations so that these lessons are not lost, but instead become our new foundation, for our country and the rest of the world, where many others learned lessons as well.

STRATEGIC LESSONS

We have learned that pandemics are an existential danger to our societies. We know that the next one could be much worse. There is a core lesson. The United States and other countries must consider how to make a profound shift, a paradigm shift, what a recent CEPI report rightly calls "a fundamental shift towards preparedness."[2]

In facing a possible pandemic, time is everything. A week can be the difference between an outbreak and an epidemic. A month can be the difference between a local epidemic and a global pandemic. This pandemic has been a planetary hit. Aside from the loss of life, its effects are still rippling through the world economy, blighting lives and intensifying conflicts, like the war in Ukraine. Throughout the Covid war, the combatants had a constant sense of being on the back foot, off balance, not ready enough.

Few will quarrel with a goal of preparedness. Governments will embrace it. Some may even issue a strategy statement.

At the start of this book, we spotlighted the importance of the "how." In that recent CEPI report, which concentrated on the "how" of the hundred-day vaccine goal, its authors used the illustration of Formula 1 racing. All the teams could see that they needed to cut the time of the pit stop, which used to take more than a minute. If well executed it now takes, at most, a few seconds.

Racing is a problem like ours, in which time is of the essence. The "how" part was not just a problem of drilling the teams. That was important, of course. But

> ultimately the transformation in pit-stop cycle times required a paradigm shift that involved redefining fundamental aspects of Formula 1, including the instrumentation for monitoring race performance, the design of the principal components of the race car and the types of tools used to maintain and change those components. This required adaptation across multiple disciplines of Formula 1, including technical research and design, development and testing, manufacturing and regulation.[3]

Pandemic preparedness is one of the few threats that genuinely deserves that intense level of attention. And this war yielded many insights about where to focus.

Real policy work is less about what "should" be done and more about how to do it, a concept of operations. The best policy work turns how-to's into routine exercises of desired capabilities.

The failure to learn the lessons the pandemic should have taught played out again in the winter of 2022–23. The United States is experiencing a healthcare crisis from the convergence of respiratory viruses—RSV, influenza, and Covid. As in 2020, the crisis was foreseen. It hit overseas before it came to the United States. As in 2020, emergency preparations to stockpile and distribute crucial medications lagged, as did practical guidance for follow-through by physicians. As in 2020, efforts to develop and distribute new tests—like "multiplex" panel screens to check a set of respiratory ailments—have faltered. As in 2020, a sagging healthcare system lacked the financial incentives or readiness to handle surges of patients, including many children. And, as in 2020, the burden of these failures falls disproportionately on stricken families and battle-weary acute caregivers.

Americans will muddle through the tripledemic, as they muddle through severe flu seasons. The healthcare system is not about to fail. But if the country can learn some of the lessons from the Covid war, Americans can do so much more to handle such events, the "normal" stresses from infectious disease, as well as the next giant outbreak. Good governments learn what to do from large emergencies and practice what they have learned in smaller ones.

We now see the need for concerned governments to develop a whole new system for governing exceptionally risky biological research. We now see the need to build up a worldwide set of early warning radars that can give enough notice of an emerging threat, a system that does not have to rely on hollow commitments from countries that may be unwilling to sound an alarm.

We see that any hope of containing an outbreak before it becomes a pandemic requires more ambitious and realistic national and international preparation. A basic requirement will be setups for biomedical surveillance that draw on our successful public-private experiments in this crisis, connecting the public health and healthcare systems. That biomedical surveillance must include ongoing gathering of evidence throughout the crisis, on how the enemy is evolving, and what defenses work best. Such readiness requires strong multinational capabilities to size up the character of the disease, quickly, even if outside experts cannot get to the site of the original outbreak (as they could not in this case) and without waiting for definitive certainties.

The frontline fighters in the Covid war have learned an enormous amount about how best to prepare for the next war. To take the example of viral threats: there are at most a few dozen families of viruses that can infect humans. It is possible to work out basic vaccine designs for each family and test ways to manufacture these designs at scale. It will take years to build out these "vaccine libraries" but then, once the specific virus has been identified in a family, the design can quickly be tailored to that version of the virus. That design can then be paired to known, proven methods for how to produce it. This is the kind of work that can turn the "vaccines in a hundred days" dream to practical possibility.

In the war we also learned more about how to prepare to produce tests at scale, and also about some of the best ways to use them in the field. We learned about the challenges of translating discoveries of new, good medicines into operational readiness so that they will actually be used, properly, in thousands of clinics or hospitals.

The war has shown us that practical preparation means advance investment and ready access to emergency funds, along with a proactive and multi-year approach to preparing partnerships with private industry to meet public needs. We also learned, again, the value of a global coalition in fighting a global war. The benefits may flow to all but, at this stage of world history, a relatively small number of countries must take on the main responsibility for organizing such a coalition. The war illustrated that, too, both for better and worse.

We have also learned a great deal about how to think about non-medical interventions in a health emergency. The United States went into this war with a concept that lockdowns might slow the spread and buy a little time. That concept was right.

But what was to come next? The prewar concepts for a lockdown assumed that, if it did not quash the outbreak, the time might be used to distribute effective medicine and clinical guidance while getting to work on the vaccine. But, in this war, the United States had trouble accurately assessing the disease, lacked effective medicine on hand to treat it, and vaccines were still a number of months away. The lockdowns could not be sustained. But leaders did not develop and communicate practical alternative strategies.

If community spread of the disease is inevitable and there are no effective medications on hand, leaders have to think hard about the practical objectives for their non-medical interventions. It is, of course, great to slow the spread. Fewer people get infected in a slower epidemic, even if rules are relaxed in the middle. Time gives doctors more of a chance to figure out how to treat the disease and spread the word. Covid patients received better treatment in November 2020 than they did in March or May. Time gets people a little closer to the availability of good drugs or vaccines.[4]

But leaders will balance those benefits against the broader social costs. The highest priority objective of the non-medical measures should be, first, to protect the most vulnerable people and the hospitals that treat them and, second, help everyone return to work or school as soon as possible without adding much more risk to the risks they already face.

The war illustrated a number of non-medical tools. The best improvisers showed that they could combine them in ways suited to the nature of the enemy and that were practical to the people who had to do the work. They helped people feel safer in returning to normal life. In this war we believe that such customized approaches became more and more feasible, at least by the autumn of 2020. This potential was not implemented quickly enough, with clear, realistic objectives in mind.

We also learned some hard lessons about the importance of crisis communication that is well considered, honest, practical, and clear. Citizens can judge for themselves how well their leaders met this standard.

LESSONS FOR INSTITUTIONS

Few things are duller to read than suggestions about how to reorganize government institutions. Also, the people running all levels of government think they know better than outsiders how to organize what they do, and they are often right.

What is most important is to specify what is to be done and have an operational conception of how to do it. Organization might, on a good day, actually follow function.

With those caveats, it is worth stressing again, as we did in chapter 3, "The Defenders," that the lessons we learned can only be applied as part of a coherent national health security enterprise. And our national effort will have to be linked globally in ways we outlined both in chapter 10 and in our chapter "Origins, Prevention, and Warning."

The national health security enterprise will need to have a focal point of operational leadership in a government department with stable appropriations. We think that department should be HHS, with the focal point a new undersecretary for health security. That executive should oversee the current assistant secretary for health (who looks after the Public Health Service), the ASPR, the CDC, and the department's office of global affairs. Only national executive leadership can orchestrate real strategies to contain an outbreak and design, produce, distribute, and deploy the toolkits of countermeasures to help communities defend themselves.

The White House is obviously important. In December 2022, the Congress legislated the creation of a new White House office outside the current domestic or national security structures. It is an Office for Pandemic Preparedness and Policy Response. Though the Biden White House had not asked for this, it will probably try to give it an important role, alongside the existing bureaucracies, including those elsewhere in the White House, already jostling for influence.

But the White House is a poor place to base the management of large operations. There is no need to harp on the role of the president in a national crisis. What is worth noticing is that the usual interagency security process, the National Security Council process, is overburdened and overextended. Meanwhile, the structure for applying science policy, the

National Science and Technology Council (NSTC), headed by the president's science adviser, is nearly moribund and little used.

In such a process, the president's science adviser would become much more important, with the kind of clout Vannevar Bush had during the Second World War. The president's science adviser might then be someone with a strong sense of how to relate science, practically, to the large work of governance, including a link to the new office for pandemic preparedness. President Biden's current science adviser, Arati Prabhakar, is someone who could do this. Reliance on NSTC-NSC may also serve America on other subjects where twenty-first-century issues are not being addressed very well by mid-twentieth-century institutions.

Our emphasis on the federal executive role is not a call for a federal monopoly on the national health security enterprise. It is a call to rebalance its management to make it more national, more operational, and less fragmented. As we pointed out in chapter 3, the current system is profoundly unbalanced.

Good biomedical surveillance, a sense of what is happening and what works, and the fielding of medical countermeasures all rely on people and organizations closest to what is going on. Federalism is an asset. The legal tools and technical systems to pool local data for national assessment are still not good enough. In August 2022, CDC director Rochelle Walensky released an agenda for "Moving Forward." It opened by declaring, "There is a strategic imperative to modernize CDC so that it consistently delivers public health information and guidance to Americans in real time." That is a fair goal. Now comes the how part.

On the front lines, we saw how the ad hoc fusion cells often put together by governors and mayors really helped bring people and their capabilities together during an emergency. These capabilities need to be regularized in peacetime, and not just in jurisdictions that experience hurricanes, fires, or tornadoes.

Executive branch policymaking, working out of Washington at the undersecretary level, will be closer to centers of federal and state leadership. In this vision, a changed CDC still has a vital role. Playing to its core strengths, CDC can track and analyze what is going on—the hub of a national network of state, local, tribal, and territorial health departments out in the field, linked to their local healthcare providers.

A SECRET OF AMERICAN GREATNESS

Americans can reflect on a proud heritage, not far in the past, when they were known across the world for their practical can-do skills in everything from fixing cars to designing European recovery to putting a man on the moon. Again and again, they tackled apparently insurmountable problems, public and private, in a get-it-done spirit. At one level the Covid crisis is another depressing story of how twenty-first-century Americans have fallen short.

Yet at another level, we show that many Americans rose to the challenge. The Covid crisis abounds with stories of desperate improvisations, in America and all over the world. Some succeeded; many failed. We hope our country will reflect on this war to prepare, not just for another pandemic, but for the kind of global emergencies that already seem to mark the twenty-first century, including changes in energy use and climate.

There are obviously several ways to explain the decline in government performance and the collapse in public trust in the U.S. government since the high-water marks of the late 1950s and early 1960s. Since the early 1960s, the government has tried to do much more, around the world and at home, and it is perceived to have often fallen short, sometimes catastrophically so.

It is not very useful to blame the anti-Washington discourse. Such scapegoating of Washington is not new. It is an old, old theme in American history. Nor should we blame incompetent delivery of basic services, which is still reasonably good in America.

Weak knowledge of the history of issues or even of the government's own policy record, a superficial grasp of other communities or institutions, and a preoccupation with reactions to daily news: these too are symptoms. They are symptoms of a weakening capacity for in-depth professional assessment.

Of course, the marked tendency to militarize policy, to rely on military instruments and military policymakers, repeated again in Operation Warp Speed, is no cure. It is another symptom of the breakdown, as American policymaking is dumbed down and becomes praetorian.

Some of these problems can be blamed on bad structures and on polarized, dysfunctional politics. But that's not all of the story. We have also learned lessons about the software of good governance.

As the immensely powerful Qing empire in China began to decay in the early 1800s, a leading scholar started calling for reform of the Confucian system that selected and trained the country's administrative elite. He looked around and saw "everything was falling apart . . . the administration was contaminated and vile." The scholar, Bao Shichen, "found himself drawn toward more practical kinds of scholarship that were not tested on the civil service exams."[5]

Bao "would in time become one of the leading figures in a field known broadly as 'statecraft' scholarship," an informal movement of Confucians who were deeply concerned with real-world issues of administration and policy. Tragically for Bao and many of his allies, their efforts were not enough. They could not reverse the decline of their empire.

The U.S. government has plenty of problems too. Fortunately, it is not yet at the point the Qing dynasty reached. Americans' seemingly bygone skills for policymaking and tackling emergencies were not in their genes or in the air. They need not be consigned to wistful nostalgia. The skills were specific. They were fostered by the surrounding culture. And they can be relearned.

ACRONYMS

ASPR	Assistant Secretary for Preparedness and Response (renamed in July 2022 to Administration for Strategic Preparedness and Response)
BARDA	Biomedical Advanced Research and Development Authority
BSL	Biosafety Level
CDC	Centers for Disease Control and Prevention
CEPI	Coalition for Epidemic Preparedness Innovations
CFA	Center for Forecasting and Outbreak Analytics
CIADM	Center for Innovation in Advanced Development and Manufacturing
CMS	Centers for Medicare and Medicaid Services
COVAX	COVID-19 Vaccines Global Access
COVID-19	Coronavirus Disease 2019
CSC	Crisis Standards of Care
DARPA	Defense Advanced Research Projects Agency
DHS	Department of Homeland Security
DPA	Defense Production Act
EUA	Emergency Use Authorization
EuroMOMO	European mortality monitoring activity
FDA	Food and Drug Administration
FEMA	Federal Emergency Management Agency
GISRS	Global Influenza Surveillance and Response System
H-CORE	HHS Coordination Operations and Response Element
HHS	Department of Health and Human Services
HRSA	Health Resources and Services Administration

KDCA	Korea Disease Control and Prevention Agency
LDT	Laboratory-Developed Test
MERS	Middle East Respiratory Syndrome
mRNA	Messenger RNA
NDMS	National Disaster Medical System
NIAID	National Institute of Allergy and Infectious Diseases
NIH	National Institutes of Health
NIOSH	National Institute for Occupational Safety and Health
NSABB	National Science Advisory Board for Biosecurity
NSC	National Security Council
OMB	Office of Management and Budget
PanCAP	Pandemic Crisis Action Plan
PCR	Polymerase Chain Reaction
PDB	President's Daily Brief
PHEMCE	Public Health Emergency Medical Countermeasures Enterprise
PHEP	Public Health Emergency Preparedness
PPE	Personal Protective Equipment
SARS	Severe Acute Respiratory Syndrome
SARS-CoV-2	Severe Acute Respiratory Syndrome Coronavirus 2
SNS	Strategic National Stockpile
USAID	United States Agency for International Development
WHO	World Health Organization

ABOUT THE COVID CRISIS GROUP

At the end of 2020, about a year into the pandemic, a group of scientists discussed the need for a national commission to learn lessons from this latest world war, against COVID-19. To them the need seemed obvious. One participant in those discussions was Eric Schmidt, the former Google executive. He had served on President Barack Obama's board of science advisors. Schmidt decided to help sponsor planning for a Covid commission. To that end, Schmidt's foundation, Schmidt Futures, helped organize a consortium with three other foundations: The Rockefeller Foundation, the Skoll Foundation, and Stand Together. Each contributed equal funds. The sponsors played no part in drafting or editing this report or its recommendations. Joining the effort was the Covid Collaborative, a group of experts and leaders in health, education, and the economy who represented the diversity of America. The Center for Health Security at Johns Hopkins University and CSIS Global Health Policy Center provided valuable support during our initial commission planning phase, as did the University of Virginia's Miller Center of Public Affairs.

The Covid Commission Planning Group turned into a Covid Crisis Group, directed by Philip Zelikow. A history professor at the University of Virginia and former official in several administrations of both parties, and leader of other commissions and study groups, he had been the executive director of the federal agency, the 9/11 Commission.

The book is truly a group project. Most people who publish in the sciences are used to working in teams. Zelikow held the pen, but every person listed below was actively involved as a co-author, even though not every author endorses every statement in the book. They contributed their views as individuals, and this book does not express the views of any institution.

The members of the group participated in the many listening sessions, which themselves became occasions for debate. They offered broad directional advice, drafted whole sections of text, debated the direction of the draft, and offered repeated comments and line edits on successive drafts.

The group had a small regular staff. Stephanie Kaplan, another veteran of the 9/11 Commission, was the chief of staff. As special assistant, Brandon Kist was a key researcher in assembling our final report; he also organized and drafted memoranda for the record for almost all of our listening sessions. Linda Listrom, a lawyer with extensive experience in complex investigations, served on the staff, as did Celeste Ward Gventer and Scott Lindsay until both returned to public service at the Department of Defense and city of Seattle, respectively. Matthew Boyce provided early research assistance.

Richard Danzig and Luciana Borio were advisers to the group and offered comments on our evolving manuscript.

In addition to Zelikow, the other members of the Covid Crisis Group are, in alphabetical order:

DANIELLE ALLEN, James Bryant Conant University Professor and Director, Edmond and Lily Safra Center for Ethics, Harvard University

JOHN M. BARRY, historian and author of *The Great Influenza: The Story of the Deadliest Pandemic in History* (2004)

JOHN BRIDGELAND, founder and CEO, COVID Collaborative, and former Director, White House Domestic Policy Council for President George W. Bush

MICHAEL CALLAHAN, staff physician, internal medicine and infectious disease, and director, clinical translation and mass casualty therapeutics, Massachusetts General Hospital

NICHOLAS A. CHRISTAKIS, physician, author of *Apollo's Arrow: The Profound and Enduring Impact of Coronavirus on the Way We Live* (2020), and director, Human Nature Lab, Yale University

DOUG CRISCITELLO, former executive director, MIT Golub Center for Finance and Policy, and former CFO, U.S. Department of Housing and Urban Development and the U.S. Small Business Administration

CHARITY DEAN, CEO and founder, The Public Health Company, and former assistant director, California Department of Public Health

VICTOR DZAU, president, National Academy of Medicine

GARY EDSON, president, COVID Collaborative, and former Deputy National Security Advisor and Deputy National Economic Advisor to President George W. Bush

EZEKIEL J. EMANUEL, vice provost for Global Initiatives and chair of the Department of Medical Ethics and Health Policy, University of Pennsylvania

RUTH FADEN, founder and Wagley Professor, Berman Institute of Bioethics, Johns Hopkins University

BARUCH FISCHHOFF, Howard Heinz University Professor, Department of Engineering & Public Policy, Institute for Politics and Strategy, Carnegie Mellon University

MARGARET "PEGGY" HAMBURG, former FDA commissioner and former New York City health commissioner

MELISSA HARVEY, Assistant Vice President, Enterprise Preparedness and Emergency Operations at HCA Healthcare

RICHARD HATCHETT, CEO, Coalition for Epidemic Preparedness Innovations (CEPI)

DAVID HEYMANN, Professor of Infectious Disease Epidemiology, London School of Hygiene and Tropical Medicine, and former Head, Centre on Global Health Security, Chatham House, London

KENDALL HOYT, Assistant Professor, Geisel School of Medicine, Senior Lecturer, Thayer School of Engineering, and Faculty Director, Pandemic Security Project at the Dickey Center, Dartmouth College

ANDREW KILIANSKI, Senior Director, Emerging Infectious Diseases, International AIDS Vaccine Initiative (IAVI), and adjunct faculty, Schar School of Policy and Government, George Mason University

JAMES LAWLER, Professor of Medicine, Division of Infectious Diseases, and Executive Director, International Programs and Innovation, Global Center for Health Security, University of Nebraska Medical Center (UNMC)

ALEXANDER J. LAZAR, Professor of Pathology & Genomic Medicine, The University of Texas MD Anderson Cancer Center

JAMES LE DUC, former director, Galveston National Laboratory, and adjunct professor, Microbiology and Immunology, University of Texas Medical Branch at Galveston

MARC LIPSITCH, Professor of Epidemiology and Director, Center for Communicable Disease Dynamics, T.H. Chan School of Public Health, Harvard University

ANUP MALANI, Lee and Brena Freeman Professor, University of Chicago Law School, and professor, Pritzker School of Medicine, University of Chicago

MONIQUE K. MANSOURA, Executive Director for Global Health Security and Biotechnology, The MITRE Corporation

MARK MCCLELLAN, former FDA commissioner, former CMS administrator, and director, Duke-Margolis Center for Health Policy, Duke University

CARTER MECHER, Medical Advisor, The Public Health Company; former Senior Medical Advisor, Office of Public Health, U.S. Department of Veterans Affairs; and former Director of Medical Preparedness Policy, White House Homeland Security Council and National Security Staff

MICHAEL OSTERHOLM, director, Center for Infectious Disease Research and Policy (CIDRAP), University of Minnesota

DAVID A. RELMAN, Thomas C. and Joan M. Merigan Professor in Medicine; Professor of Microbiology & Immunology at Stanford University School of Medicine;

and Senior Fellow at the Freeman Spogli Institute for
International Studies at Stanford University

ROBERT RODRIGUEZ, professor of emergency medicine,
University of California, San Francisco (UCSF) School of
Medicine

CARL SCHRAMM, University Professor, Syracuse University

EMILY SILVERMAN, Assistant Volunteer Professor of
Medicine, University of California, San Francisco (UCSF)
School of Medicine, and founder/host of *The Nocturnists*

KRISTIN URQUIZA, co-founder, Marked By COVID

RAJEEV VENKAYYA, CEO, Aerium Therapeutics and former
Special Assistant to the President for Biodefense

SOURCES

Our group began its work as the Covid Commission Planning Group in February 2021. In preparation for a possible commission, we held 195 listening sessions with 274 participants. These sessions encompassed a broad spectrum of experts on the Covid crisis, including physicians, scientists, survivors and advocacy groups, public health experts, economists, academics, business executives, federal, state, and local government officials, congressional leaders and staff, and many others. Most of these sessions took place in 2021 and early 2022 over videoconference. Almost all were then summarized in memoranda for the record. We will deposit these and other materials as historical records.

The people we talked to are listed below. This is just a sample of the people we could, and perhaps should, have spoken with.

While we were conducting these listening sessions, our group organized task forces to conduct background research. In the first phase, in the first half of 2021, we obtained valuable research support from experts in the Center for Health Security at Johns Hopkins University and in the Global Health Policy Center at the Center for Strategic and International Studies. In our next phase, in the rest of 2021 and on into 2022, we organized into task forces that developed scope papers, held a number of group discussions, and gathered twice, in person, to discuss and refine the work.

We have looked at several congressional reports about the crisis. We found it quite valuable to supplement our own listening sessions with the transcribed interviews of a number of leading officials conducted in late 2021 and 2022 by majority and minority staff of the House Select Subcommittee on the Coronavirus Crisis. These were not public hearings, but some of these transcribed interviews have been made public. We also welcomed and benefited from the strong investigative work into the organization of federal crisis management in the early months of the crisis by the majority staff of the Senate Homeland Security and Governmental Affairs Committee.

Danielle Allen
American Nurses Association (3)
American Pharmacists
    Association (3)
Lloyd Armbrust
Mara Aspinall
Association of State and
    Territorial Health
    Officials (3)
John M. Barry
Trevor Bedford
Georges Benjamin
Carl Bergstrom
Ruth Bernheim
Richard Besser
Jay Bhattacharya
Paul Biddinger
Biosecurity Analysis Seminar (7)
Patrick Blair
Jesse Bloom
Timothy Blute
Body Politic (3)
Thomas Bollyky

Luciana Borio
Chad Bown
Rick Bright
Larry Brilliant
Susan Brooks
Sylvia Mathews Burwell
Michael Callahan
Michael Carney
Daniel Carpenter
Rocco Casagrande
Alina Chan
Nicholas A. Christakis
Christopher Chute
Sara Cody
Rita Colwell
Yvonne Commodore-Mensah
Lisa Cooper
Brooke Courtney
COVID Collaborative (2)
The COVID Tracking
    Project (3)
Tyler Cowen
Nancy Cox

Doug Criscitello
Glenn Cross
CSIS Commission on
   Strengthening America's
   Health Security (11)
Mitch Daniels
Richard Danzig
Natalie Davis
Charity Dean
Nancy-Ann DeParle
Philip Dormitzer
Victor Dzau
Ezekiel J. Emanuel
Drew Erdmann
Stephen Eubank
Ruth Faden
Jeremy Farrar
Anthony Fauci
Mark Ferguson
Niall Ferguson
Harvey Fineberg
Baruch Fischhoff
David Franz
Tom Frieden
Bill Frist
Sandro Galea
Atul Gawande
Helene Gayle
Bruce Gellin
Dylan George
Julie Gerberding
Eric Goosby
Celine Gounder

Ellie Graeden
Christine Gregoire
Joseph Grogan
Gigi Gronvall
Sunetra Gupta
Peter Haaland
Margaret Hamburg
Harvard Medical School
   Program in Global Public
   Policy and Social Change (3)
Melissa Harvey
Richard Hatchett
Healthcare Leadership
   Council (5)
Matthew Hepburn
David Heymann
Jane Hopkins
Kendall Hoyt
Nathaniel Hupert
Asa Hutchinson
Thomas Inglesby
John Ioannidis
Ashish Jha
Simon Johnson
Robert Kadlec
Norm Kahn
Rebecca Katz
Gerald Keusch
Andrew Kilianski
Christopher Kirchhoff
Albert Ko
Florian Krammer
Adam Kucharski

Christopher Lake
Eric Lander
Thomas LaVeist
James Lawler
Marcelle Layton
Alexander J. Lazar
James Le Duc
Michael Leavitt
Jeffrey Levi
Michael Lewis
Ian Lipkin
Marc Lipsitch
Long Haul COVID
    Fighters (3)
Nicole Lurie
Anup Malani
Monique K. Mansoura
Marked By Covid (2)
Howard Markel
Peter Marks
John Marr
Stephanie Mayfield
Bill McBride
Maureen McCarthy
McChrystal Group (9)
Mark McClellan
Matthew McGarrity
Christian McMillen
Carter Mecher
Nancy Messonnier
Lauren Ancel Meyers
David Michaels
Maureen Miller

Michael Mina
Judy Monroe
Julie Morita
John Muckstadt
Christopher Murray
National Association of County
    and City Health Officials (5)
New York City COVID-19 Oral
    History, Narrative and
    Memory Archive (4)
Indra Nooyi
Anders Nordstrom
Jennifer Nuzzo
David O'Connor
Emily Oster
Michael Osterholm
Tara O'Toole
Anand Parekh
Patient-Led Research
    Collaborative (3)
Gustave Perna
David Persse
Matthew Pottinger
President Barack Obama's
    Council of Advisors on
    Science and Technology (7)
Jonathan Quick
Jason Rao
Sarah Ratcliffe
Stephen Redd
David A. Relman
Caitlin Rivers
Robert Rodriguez

Paul Romer
Roni Rosenfeld
Marguerite Roza
Jay Schnitzer
Carl Schramm
Anne Schuchat
Kathleen Sebelius
Nirav Shah
Josh Sharfstein
Emily Silverman
Stewart Simonson
Moncef Slaoui
Andy Slavitt
Janice Stein
Jake Sullivan
Survivor Corps (4)
Andrew Sweet
Alex Tabarrok
Eric Toner
Eric Topol
Tevi Troy
Reed Tuckson
Sylvester Turner
U.S. House Committee on
    Science, Space &

Technology, Investigations
    Subcommittee Majority
    Staff (3)
U.S. House Permanent Select
    Committee on Intelligence
    Majority Staff (2)
U.S. Senate Committee on
    Health, Education, Labor
    and Pensions Majority
    Staff (3)
UNICEF (4)
Patrick Vallance
Rajeev Venkayya
Michael Watson
Clint Watts
Richard Webby
Leana Wen
Ed Whiting
Stephen Williams
James Wilson
Ngaire Woods
Michael Worobey
Lawrence Wright
Anne Wyllie
Kevin Yeskey

Quotations that are not attributed in the notes derive from listening sessions, task force meetings, and other outreach performed by our group.

NOTES

CHAPTER 1. FROM TRAGEDY TO POSSIBILITY

1. One of the classic works on historical pandemics is William H. McNeill, *Plagues and Peoples* (New York: Anchor Books, 1976); a recent distillation with a careful bibliography is Christian W. McMillen, *Pandemics: A Very Short Introduction* (New York: Oxford University Press, 2016). The definitive account of the 1918–19 influenza pandemic, at least for the United States experience, is John M. Barry, *The Great Influenza: The Epic Story of the Deadliest Plague in History* (New York: Viking Penguin, 2004). For a good overview of the historical context and societal implications of COVID-19 see Nicholas A. Christakis, *Apollo's Arrow: The Profound and Enduring Impact of Coronavirus on the Way We Live* (New York: Little, Brown Spark, 2020). An early focus on American state capacity was Brink Lindsey, "Incapacitated: How a Lack of State Capacity Doomed Pandemic Results," Niskanen Center State Capacity Project, October 24, 2022 (online). For more on the "software" of public problem-solving see Philip Zelikow, "To Regain Policy Competence: The Software of American Public Problem-Solving," *Texas National Security Review* 2, no. 4 (September 2019): 110–127.

2. One early effort to compare infection fatality rates (IFRs) from COVID-19 to the 1918 influenza arrived at a rough estimate of an 0.5 percent IFR for COVID-19 and a 2 percent IFR for the 1918 influenza, implying the latter was four times more lethal. See Daihai He et al., "Comparing COVID-19 and the 1918–19 Influenza Pandemics in the United Kingdom," *International Journal of Infectious Diseases* 98 (September 2020): 67–70.

3. For a comparison of SARS-CoV-1 and SARS-CoV-2 see Nicholas Christakis, "Nicholas Christakis on Fighting Covid-19 by Truly Understanding the Virus," *Economist*, August 10, 2020 (online).

4. "Trump was a comorbidity" came from one of our group members in a 2021 discussion. Michael Lewis also heard the same expression from one of his sources, quoted in the prologue of *The Premonition: A Pandemic Story* (New York: Norton, 2021).

5. Global and U.S. premature death figures are sourced from the *Economist*'s excess death estimates. See "The Pandemic's True Death Toll," *Economist,* updated October 25, 2022 (online). For one-third were young or middle-age, see "Excess Deaths Associated with COVID-19," Centers for Disease Control and Prevention dashboard and dataset, updated January 4, 2023 (online). The United States suffered a drop in life expectancy larger than the drop it suffered during the Second World War, see Jonas Schöley et al., "Life Expectancy Changes Since COVID-19," *Nature Human Behaviour,* October 17, 2022 (online).

6. Hospitalization number is based on data from the CDC's "COVID Data Tracker" and estimates provided in Alexia Couture et al., "Estimating COVID-19 Hospitalizations in the United States with Surveillance Data Using a Bayesian Hierarchical Model: Modeling Study," *JMIR Public Health and Surveillance* 8, no. 6 (June 2022): 34296. For Covid's impact on the elderly see "Hospitalization and Death by Age," Centers for Disease Control and Prevention, updated September 16, 2022 (online); on rural communities see Lauren Weber, "Covid Is Killing Rural Americans at Twice the Rate of Urbanites," *Kaiser Health News,* September 30, 2021 (online); on racial minorities see Latoya Hill and Samantha Artiga, "COVID-19 Cases and Deaths by Race/Ethnicity: Current Data and Changes over Time," Kaiser Family Foundation brief, August 22, 2022 (online).

7. For excess mortality data and analysis see Lauren M. Rossen et al., "Excess All-Cause Mortality in the USA and Europe during the COVID-19 Pandemic, 2020 and 2021," *Scientific Reports* 12, no. 1 (November 2022): 18559; "Excess Deaths Associated with COVID-19," CDC, updated January 4, 2023 (online); "Global Excess Deaths Associated with COVID-19, January 2020–December 2021," World Health Organization summary and dataset, May 2022 (online); and "The Pandemic's True Death Toll," *Economist,* updated October 25, 2022 (online).

8. In 2020, the median age for the United States was 37.5 years and for the EuroMOMO group it was 41.5 years. For country median age data see United Nations, Department of Economic and Social Affairs, Population Division, *World Population Prospects 2022,* 2022 (online). For Florida's median age see "New Census Bureau Visualization Shows Broad Variations in Age Structure by State and County," United States Census Bureau, July 19, 2022 (online). For the significance of median age in COVID-19 mortality see Xue-Qiang Wang et al., "Association between Aging

Population, Median Age, Life Expectancy and Mortality in Coronavirus Disease (COVID-19)," *Aging* 12, no. 24 (November 2020): 24570–24578.

9. For 391,000 fewer deaths see Rossen et al., "Excess All-Cause Mortality in the USA and Europe during the COVID-19 Pandemic, 2020 and 2021." A difficulty in comparing all-cause mortality is that there may be some additional causes in the United States that aren't entirely related to COVID-19, such as overdose and firearm-related deaths. One study estimates excess overdose mortality in 2020 at 7,600; see Abigail R. Cartus et al., "Forecasted and Observed Drug Overdose Deaths in the US During the COVID-19 Pandemic in 2020," *JAMA Network Open* 5, no. 3 (March 2022): 223418. Another study estimates that there were over four thousand excess deaths from firearm violence in 2020; see Shengzhi Sun et al., "Analysis of Firearm Violence during the COVID-19 Pandemic in the US," *JAMA Network Open* 5, no. 4 (April 2022): 229393. This, too, is part of a pattern of the pandemic exacerbating all the other prevailing ills. According to the U.S. Department of Veterans Affairs, U.S. service member deaths in World War II were 405,399. See Department of Veterans Affairs, "America's Wars," VA Office of Public Affairs, May 2021 (online).

The differential in excess deaths estimate comes from analysis of mortality rates and vaccine and booster uptake between the United States and EuroMOMO countries in 2022. See "Cumulative Confirmed COVID-19 Deaths per Million People," *Our World in Data*, accessed November 13, 2022 (online) and "COVID-19 Vaccine Booster Administered per 100 People," *Our World in Data*, accessed November 13, 2022 (online).

10. For the $5 trillion estimate see Congressional Budget Office, *The Budgetary Effects of Laws Enacted in Response to the 2020 Coronavirus Pandemic, March and April 2020*, June 2020 (online) and Congressional Budget Office, *The Budgetary Effects of Major Laws Enacted in Response to the 2020–2021 Coronavirus Pandemic, December 2020 and March 2021*, September 2021 (online).

11. Bryan W. Roberts, "The Macroeconomic Impacts of the 9/11 Attack: Evidence from Real-Time Forecasting," Department of Homeland Security working paper, August 2009 (online).

12. David M. Cutler and Lawrence H. Summers, "The COVID-19 Pandemic and the $16 Trillion Virus," *JAMA* 324, no. 15 (October 2020): 1495–1496.

13. For "spending billions to save trillions" see Susan Athey et al., "Expanding Capacity for Vaccines against COVID-19 and Future Pandemics: A Review of Economic Issues," National Bureau of Economic

Research working paper, July 2022, 25 (online). For the cost of Operation Warp Speed see Congressional Research Service, "The U.S. Government's Role in Domestic and Global COVID-19 Vaccine Supply and Distribution: Frequently Asked Questions," February 17, 2022 (online).

14. Johns Hopkins Center for Health Security, *Global Health Security Index,* October 2019 (online).

15. Fareed Zakaria, *Ten Lessons for a Post-Pandemic World* (New York: W.W. Norton, digital ed. 2020), 29.

16. Adam Taylor, "How the $1.9 Trillion U.S. Stimulus Package Compares with Other Countries' Coronavirus Spending," *Washington Post,* April 5, 2021 (online).

17. See He et al., "Comparing COVID-19 and the 1918–19 Influenza Pandemics in the United Kingdom," 67–70.

18. Quotes from Zakaria, *Ten Lessons for a Post-Pandemic World,* 28–29 (digital).

19. George Marshall radio address, April 1947, quoted in Philip Zelikow, "George C. Marshall and the Moscow CFM Meeting of 1947," *Diplomacy and Statecraft* 8, no. 2 (1997): 97, 116.

20. Michael Lewis, *The Fifth Risk* (New York: W.W. Norton, digital ed. 2018), 25–26.

21. Lewis, *The Fifth Risk,* 24 (digital).

22. Deborah Birx, *Silent Invasion: The Untold Story of the Trump Administration, Covid-19, and Preventing the Next Pandemic Before It's Too Late* (New York: Harper, digital ed. 2022), 153.

23. See John M. Barry, *Rising Tide: The Great Mississippi Flood of 1927 and How It Changed America* (New York: Simon & Schuster, 1997).

24. Ariana Eunjung Cha, "10.5 Million Children Lost a Parent or Caregiver Because of Covid, Study Says," *Washington Post,* September 6, 2022 (online).

25. For more on the experience of Long Covid see Fiona Lowenstein, ed., *The Long COVID Survival Guide: How to Take Care of Yourself and What Comes Next—Stories and Advice from Twenty Long-Haulers and Experts* (New York: The Experiment, 2022). For the costs of Long Covid see David M. Cutler, "The Costs of Long COVID," *JAMA Health Forum* 3, no. 5 (May 2022): 221809.

26. One bill to create a commission cleared committee in the Senate by a wide bipartisan margin in March 2022 but never got a floor vote. "HELP Committee Passes Murray-Burr PREVENT Pandemics Act in Overwhelming Bipartisan Vote," U.S. Senate Committee on Health, Education,

Labor, and Pensions press release, March 15, 2022 (online); Washington Post Editorial Board, "Congress Has Not Stepped Up to Fight Covid-19— or the Next Pandemic," *Washington Post*, January 8, 2023 (online).

27. The full quote from Kingdon reads: "There is a difference between a condition and a problem. We put up with all manner of conditions every day: bad weather, unavoidable and untreatable illnesses, pestilence, poverty, fanaticism. . . . Conditions become defined as problems when we come to believe that we should do something about them." From John W. Kingdon, *Agendas, Alternatives, and Public Policies* (Boston: Little, Brown, 1984), 115.

CHAPTER 2. ORIGINS, PREVENTION, AND WARNING

1. Among the books and articles already published on the origins of the COVID-19 pandemic, some contrasting views are ably explained in Martin Enserink, "'Lab-leak' and Natural Origin Proponents Face Off— Civilly—in Forum on Pandemic Origins," *Science* (with associated video), September 30, 2021 (online); Nicholas Wade, "The Origin of COVID: Did People or Nature Open Pandora's Box at Wuhan?" *Bulletin of the Atomic Scientists*, May 5, 2021 (online); David Quammen, *Breathless: The Scientific Race to Defeat a Deadly Virus* (New York: Simon & Schuster, digital ed. 2022), chapters 60–71; and Jeremy Farrar and Anjana Ahuja, *Spike: The Virus vs. The People—The Inside Story* (London: Profile Books, digital ed. 2021), chapters 2–3. For background on the proliferation of labs doing high-risk research see Smriti Mallapaty, "COVID Prompts Global Surge in Labs That Handle Dangerous Pathogens," *Nature*, October 11, 2022 (online). On efforts to govern the most risky research see Jocelyn Kaiser, "Making Trouble," *Science*, October 19, 2022 (online), and Jaspreet Pannu et al., "Strengthen Oversight of Risky Research on Pathogens," *Science* 378, no. 6625 (December 2022): 1170–1172. On the clandestine Soviet biological weapons program see Milton Leitenberg and Raymond Zilinskas, *The Soviet Biological Weapons Program: A History* (Cambridge, MA: Harvard University Press, 2012) and David Hoffman, *The Dead Hand* (New York: Doubleday, 2009).

For the emergence of SARS-CoV-1 see David Cyranoski, "Bat Cave Solves Mystery of Deadly SARS Virus—and Suggests New Outbreak Could Occur," *Nature*, December 1, 2017 (online).

2. David Stanway, "Explainer: China's Mojiang Mine and Its Role in the Origins of COVID-19," *Reuters*, June 9, 2021 (online).

3. Denise Grady, "Camels Linked to Spread of MERS Virus in People," *New York Times*, February 25, 2014 (online).

4. Peter Li, "Reopening the Trade after SARS: China's Wildlife Industry and the Fateful Policy Reversal," *Environmental Policy and Law* 50, no. 3 (December 2020): 251–267.

5. Michael Worobey et al., "The Huanan Seafood Wholesale Market in Wuhan Was the Early Epicenter of the COVID-19 Pandemic," *Science* 377, no. 6609 (July 2022): 951–959.

6. Chen Wang et al., "A Novel Coronavirus Outbreak of Global Health Concern," *Lancet* 395, no. 10223 (February 2020): 470–473.

7. Jonathan E. Pekar et al., "The Molecular Epidemiology of Multiple Zoonotic Origins of SARS-CoV-2," *Science* 377, no. 6609 (July 2022): 960–966.

8. Edward C. Holmes et al., "The Origins of SARS-CoV-2: A Critical Review," *Cell* 184, no. 19 (September 2021): 4848–4856.

9. Jayson S. Jia et al., "Population Flow Drives Spatio-Temporal Distribution of COVID-19 in China," *Nature* 582, no. 7812 (April 2020): 389–394.

10. Jon Cohen, "Anywhere But Here," *Science*, August 18, 2022 (online).

11. Dennis Normile, "Mounting Lab Miscues Raise SARS Fears," *Science*, April 27, 2004 (online).

12. For NSABB proposed guidelines see National Science Advisory Board for Biosecurity, *Recommendations for the Evaluation and Oversight of Proposed Gain-of-Function Research*, May 2016 (online). For HHS-sponsored work see U.S. Department of Health and Human Services, *Framework for Guiding Funding Decisions about Proposed Research Involving Enhanced Potential Pandemic Pathogens*, 2017 (online).

13. Dake Kang et al., "China Clamps Down in Hidden Hunt for Coronavirus Origins," *AP*, December 30, 2020 (online); Eva Dou, "Wuhan Lab's Classified Work Complicates Search for Pandemic's Origins," *Washington Post*, June 22, 2021 (online).

14. Scott Shane, "F.B.I., Laying Out Evidence, Closes Anthrax Case," *New York Times*, February 19, 2010 (online).

15. Filippa Lentzos and Gregory Koblentz, "Fifty-nine Labs around World Handle the Deadliest Pathogens—Only a Quarter Score High on Safety," *Conversation*, June 14, 2021 (online).

16. For agencies of the U.S. government see Sharon Lerner et al., "NIH Documents Provide New Evidence U.S. Funded Gain-of-Function Research in Wuhan," *Intercept*, September 9, 2021 (online).

17. Sheri Fink and Mike Baker, "'It's Just Everywhere Already': How Delays in Testing Set Back the U.S. Coronavirus Response," *New York Times*, March 10, 2020 (online).

18. James Gorman, "China's Ban on Wildlife Trade a Big Step, but Has Loopholes, Conservationists Say," *New York Times*, February 27, 2020 (online).

19. The 2019-nCoV Outbreak Joint Field Epidemiology Investigation Team, "An Outbreak of NCIP (2019-NCoV) Infection in China—Wuhan, Hubei Province, 2019–2020," *China CDC Weekly* 2, no. 5 (January 2020): 79–80; Chaolin Huang et al., "Clinical Features of Patients Infected with 2019 Novel Coronavirus in Wuhan, China," *Lancet* 395, no. 10223 (February 2020): 497–506.

20. Ewen Callaway, "China Coronavirus: Labs Worldwide Scramble to Analyse Live Samples," *Nature*, January 31, 2020 (online).

21. For more on the bio revolution see Michael Chui et al., *The Bio Revolution: Innovations Transforming Economies, Societies, and Our Lives*, McKinsey Global Institute, May 13, 2020 (online).

22. For details on the disclosure of the Soviet biological weapons program and subsequent diplomacy see Philip Zelikow and Condoleezza Rice, *To Build a Better World: Choices to End the Cold War and Create a Global Commonwealth* (New York: Twelve, 2019), 258–262, 316, 327.

23. On the clandestine Soviet biological weapons program see Leitenberg and Zilinskas, *The Soviet Biological Weapons Program* and Hoffman, *The Dead Hand*.

24. Charles Perrow, *Normal Accidents: Living with High-Risk Technologies* (New York: Basic Books, 1984).

25. Paul Berg, "Asilomar 1975: DNA Modification Secured," *Nature* 455, no. 7211 (September 2008): 290–291.

26. Georgios Pappas, "The Lanzhou Brucella Leak: The Largest Laboratory Accident in the History of Infectious Diseases?" *Clinical Infectious Diseases* 75, no. 10 (November 2022): 1845–1847. For biosafety laws see Sally Huang, "Commentary—Assessing China's New Biosafety Law," *Pandora Report*, produced by the George Mason University Schar School of Policy and Government biodefense program, March 19, 2021 (online). For U.S. concerns about biosafety and corruption, see, e.g., Denise Grady, "Deadly Germ Research Is Shut Down at Army Lab Over Safety Concerns," *New*

York Times, August 5, 2019 (online); Heather Moniglio, "CDC Inspection Findings Reveal More about USAMRID Research Suspension," *Frederick News-Post*, November 23, 2019 (online); Dave Kovaleski, "Maryland Lawmakers Applaud CDC's Decision to Reopen Fort Detrick Facility," *Homeland Preparedness News*, April 1, 2020 (online).

CHAPTER 3. THE DEFENDERS

1. A good overview of the development of the public health profession in the United States can be found in Elizabeth Fee, *Disease and Discovery: A History of the Johns Hopkins School of Hygiene and Public Health, 1916–1939* (Baltimore: Johns Hopkins University Press, 1987), chapter 1. For an overview of the variation in U.S. local health departments see National Association of County and City Health Officials, *National Profile of Local Health Departments*, 2019 (online). For a deep dive into the world of local public health officers see Michael Lewis, *The Premonition* (New York: W.W. Norton, digital ed. 2021), chapter 2. For background on the U.S. pandemic preparedness efforts in the early 2000s see Lewis, *The Premonition*, chapters 3–5. For proposed reforms to the American public health system see the Commonwealth Fund Commission on a National Public Health System, *Meeting America's Public Health Challenge: Recommendations for Building a National Public Health System That Addresses Ongoing and Future Health Crises, Advances Equity, and Earns Trust*, June 2022 (online).

Quote, from bacteriologist William Sedgwick, found in Fee, *Disease and Discovery*, chapter 1.

2. For discussion of the public health eras and source for the "health, equity, and resilience in communities" quote see Karen B. DeSalvo et al., "Public Health 3.0: A Call to Action for Public Health to Meet the Challenges of the 21st Century," *Preventing Chronic Disease* 14 (September 2017): 170017.

3. For background on community health workers see Shreya Kangovi and Uché Blackstock, "Community Health Workers Are Essential in This Crisis. We Need More of Them," *Washington Post*, July 3, 2020 (online) and Ed Yong, "America Is Sliding into the Long Pandemic Defeat," *Atlantic*, June 27, 2022 (online).

4. In 2021, federally qualified health centers, also known as community health centers, served 30 million Americans. For data on these health

centers see "America's Health Centers," an infographic produced by the National Association of Community Health Centers, August 2022 (online).

5. For quotes from Anne Schuchat see Council of State and Territorial Epidemiologists, *Driving Public Health in the Fast Lane: The Urgent Need for a 21st Century Data Superhighway*, September 2019, 8 (online). For "manual paper-based methods" and "vast disconnect" quotes see Council of State and Territorial Epidemiologists, *Driving Public Health in the Fast Lane*, 10.

6. Quote from Rochelle Walensky in Sharon LaFraniere, "'Very Harmful' Lack of Data Blunts U.S. Response to Outbreaks," *New York Times*, September 20, 2022 (online).

7. For public health staffing and funding shortages see the Commonwealth Fund Commission on a National Public Health System, *Meeting America's Public Health Challenge*, 11.

8. For Robert Redfield quotes see U.S. House of Representatives Select Subcommittee on the Coronavirus Crisis, "Interview of Robert Redfield," March 17, 2022, 208–210 (online).

9. For Brett Giroir quotes see U.S. House of Representatives Select Subcommittee on the Coronavirus Crisis, "Interview of Brett Giroir," May 3, 2022, 153–156 (online).

10. Select Subcommittee on the Coronavirus Crisis, "Interview of Robert Redfield," 66.

11. Partnership for Public Service, Samuel J. Heyman Service to America Medals honoree profile for Anita Patel, 2022 (online). For details on the creation of public-private partnerships with pharmacy companies to deliver vaccines see Paul Mango, *Warp Speed: Inside the Operation That Beat COVID, the Critics, and the Odds* (New York: Republic, digital ed. 2022), 109–110.

12. For quotes from Anne Schuchat see U.S. House of Representatives Select Subcommittee on the Coronavirus Crisis, "Interview of Anne Schuchat," October 1, 2021, 85–87 (online).

13. Lewis, *The Premonition*, 53 (digital).

14. U.S. Department of Health and Human Services, *2012 Public Health Emergency Medical Countermeasures Enterprise (PHEMCE) Strategy*, 2012, 22 (online).

15. On the $29 billion, see Office of Management and Budget, *The Budget for Fiscal Year 2021*, Budget Appendix, 548. For more on FEMA authorities and flexibility, see Majority Staff of U.S. Senate Committee on

Homeland Security and Governmental Affairs, *Historically Unprepared: Examination of the Federal Government's COVID-19 Pandemic Preparedness and Response*, December 2022 (online) (hereinafter referred to as Senate HSGA Majority Staff, *Examination*).

16. Scott Gottlieb, *Uncontrolled Spread: Why COVID-19 Crushed Us and How We Can Defeat the Next Pandemic* (New York: Harper, digital ed. 2021), 160.

17. For background on this fund see Alison Kodjak, "A Permanent Fund That Could Help Fight Zika Exists, but It's Empty," *NPR*, June 3, 2016 (online) and Jennifer B. Alton and Ellen P. Carlin, "Now Is the Time to Resource the Public Health Emergency Fund," *Hill*, February 28, 2020 (online). The Public Health Emergency Fund is federal account #075-1104, and its historical balances can be found at www.usaspending.gov.

18. For details on this fund see Alton and Carlin, "Now Is the Time to Resource the Public Health Emergency Fund; see also, including for the $105 million figure, Senate HSGA Majority Staff, *Examination*, Table 3, 43.

19. President Donald J. Trump, Executive Order 13887, "Modernizing Influenza Vaccines in the United States to Promote National Security and Public Health," September 19, 2019.

20. "Immediate action" quote from Executive Office of the President, Letter from the President's Council of Advisors on Science and Technology to President Barack Obama, November 2016 (online).

21. White House official quotes are from Ronald Klain, "Confronting the Pandemic Threat," *Democracy: A Journal of Ideas*, no. 40 (Spring 2016) (online).

22. Executive Office of the President, Council of Economic Advisers, *Mitigating the Impact of Pandemic Influenza through Vaccine Innovation*, September 2019, 1 (online).

23. "Evolution of Biodefense Policy," Robert Strauss Center YouTube video, October 18, 2018 (online).

CHAPTER 4. CONTAINMENT FAILS; MOBILIZATION LAGS

1. For U.S. containment, testing and data failures see Lawrence Wright, *The Plague Year: America in the Time of Covid* (New York: Alfred A. Knopf, digital ed. 2021), chapters 1–12; Gottlieb, *Uncontrolled Spread*, chapters 1–13; Birx, *Silent Invasion*, chapters 1–10; Lewis, *The Premonition*, chapters

7–10. For background on South Korea's response to the pandemic see June-Ho Kim et al., "Emerging COVID-19 Success Story: South Korea Learned the Lessons of MERS," *Exemplars in Global Health*, March 5, 2021 (online); for contrast between the South Korean and U.S. testing approaches see U.S. Food and Drug Administration Center for Devices and Radiological Health, *South Korea's Response to COVID-19*, May 27, 2021 (online) and Gottlieb, *Uncontrolled Spread*, chapter 14. For background on Germany's response to the pandemic see Lothar Wieler et al., "Emerging COVID-19 Success Story: Germany's Push to Maintain Progress," *Exemplars in Global Health*, March 20, 2021 (online).

For Sharfstein book quote see Joshua Sharfstein, *The Public Health Crisis Survival Guide: Leadership and Management in Trying Times* (New York: Oxford University Press, 2018), 62. Though not one of the co-authors of this book, Sharfstein was a frequent adviser in our efforts.

2. Our half-dozen begins with Yasmeen Abutaleb & Damian Paletta, *Nightmare Scenario: Inside the Trump Administration's Response to the Pandemic That Changed History* (New York: Harper, digital ed. 2022); Wright, *The Plague Year*; Bob Woodward, *Rage* (New York: Simon & Schuster, 2020); Brendan Borrell, *The First Shots: The Epic Rivalries and Heroic Science behind the Race to the Coronavirus Vaccine* (Boston: Mariner Books, digital ed. 2021); Peter Baker & Susan Glasser, *The Divider: Trump in the White House, 2017–2021* (New York: Doubleday, 2022); and Gottlieb, *Uncontrolled Spread*. Unless we use direct quotations, or otherwise cite a source, our discussion of the arguments in the Trump administration in this early period are drawn from these published sources and our listening sessions with several of those involved, who are listed at the front of this section.

3. For details on Jeremy Farrar's calls with George Gao see Farrar and Ahuja, *Spike*, 6.

4. For Robert Redfield's calls with George Gao and Tedros Adhanom Ghebreyesus see Select Subcommittee on the Coronavirus Crisis, "Interview of Robert Redfield," 20–25.

5. For additional background on the Wolverines see Lewis, *The Premonition*, chapter 7 (digital).

6. We talked to Bright, and parts of his account, including the exchanges with Mike Bowen at Prestige Ameritech, can be corroborated from email chains he supplied as exhibits to the whistleblower complaint he filed in May 2020, after leaving the government (available online). See also Wright, *The Plague Year*, 42–43. On Osterholm and 3M's preparations,

see David Freedman, "How 3M Blew Its Reputation on the N95 Mask," *Marker-Medium*, August 19, 2020 (online).

7. Farrar and Ahuja, *Spike*, 26 (digital).

8. Farrar and Ahuja, *Spike*, 48 (digital).

9. For more on Pottinger see Wright, *The Plague Year*, 12–13, 61–62 (digital).

10. Borio has been a frequent adviser to our group and, at FDA, worked for a member of our group, Peggy Hamburg.

11. Quotes from the PDB session are from Pottinger and Woodward, *Rage*, xiii–xv, who identifies Sanner as the briefer. Sanner has discussed her service publicly. See Luciana Borio and Scott Gottlieb, "Act Now to Prevent an American Epidemic," *Wall Street Journal*, January 28, 2020 (online). For the Callahan report, Borrell, *The First Shots*, 51 [digital].

12. On Mulvaney, Baker and Glasser, *The Divider*, 418–419 (digital), quoting Navarro memo, "Impose Travel Ban on China," January 29, 2020. It is hard to tell, in this memo or later ones, how Navarro arrived at his cost and mortality estimates.

13. For information on the successes and failures of intelligence gathering early in the pandemic, see Majority Staff of U.S. House of Representatives Permanent Select Committee on Intelligence, *Declassified Report Examining the Intelligence Community's Response to the COVID-19 Pandemic*, December 15, 2022 (online).

14. Bob Woodward, *The Trump Tapes* (New York: Simon & Schuster, 2022, audiobook), Interview #7 and Interview #9.

15. For an early example of media coverage about the pandemic playbook, and a link to a PDF of the playbook, see Dan Diamond and Nahal Toosi, "Trump Team Failed to Follow NSC's Pandemic Playbook," *Politico*, March 25, 2020 (online).

16. "Kitty cat" quote is from Abutaleb and Paletta, *Nightmare Scenario*, 60 (digital).

17. Select Subcommittee on the Coronavirus Crisis, "Interview of Brett Giroir," 22.

18. Select Subcommittee on the Coronavirus Crisis, "Interview of Brett Giroir," 44.

19. David Morgan et al., "Understanding Differences in Health Expenditure between the United States and OECD Countries," Organisation for Economic Co-operation and Development, September 2022 (online).

20. For debates within the U.S. Government about travel bans see Wright, *Plague Year*, 59-61, 111–115.

21. Matteo Chinazzi et al., "The Effect of Travel Restrictions on the Spread of the 2019 Novel Coronavirus (COVID-19) Outbreak," *Science* 368, no. 6489 (March 2020): 395–400.

22. For background on COVID-NET see Center for Disease Control and Prevention, "Coronavirus Disease 2019 (COVID-19)-Associated Hospitalization Surveillance Network (COVID-NET)," updated September 9, 2022 (online).

23. For background on NIH investment in biocontainment labs see James W. Le Duc, "Biocontainment Laboratories: A Critical Component of the US Bioeconomy in Need of Attention," *Health Security* 18, no. 1 (February 2020): 61–66.

24. "CDC Statement on COVID-19 Apple App," CDC press release, March 27, 2020 (online).

25. Birx, *Silent Invasion*, 28–29 (digital).

26. Joseph A. Lewnard et al., "Clinical Outcomes Associated with SARS-CoV-2 Omicron (B.1.1.529) Variant and BA.1/BA.1.1 or BA.2 Subvariant Infection in Southern California," *Nature Medicine* 28, no. 9 (June 2022): 1933–1943.

27. For a timeline of testing events from January to May 2020 see Suzanne Murrin, *FDA Repeatedly Adapted Emergency Use Authorization Policies to Address the Need for COVID-19 Testing*, U.S. Department of Health and Human Services Office of Inspector General, September 2022, 8 (online).

28. Abutaleb and Paletta, *Nightmare Scenario*, 255–256 (digital).

CHAPTER 5. FEDERAL CRISIS MANAGEMENT COLLAPSES; OPERATION WARP SPEED BEGINS

1. On Crimson Contagion see, for example, David E. Sanger et al., "Before Virus Outbreak, a Cascade of Warnings Went Unheeded," *New York Times*, March 19, 2020 (online). On the breakdown of federal crisis management and overreliance on the influenza model see Birx, *Silent Invasion*, chapters 8–10; Gottlieb, *Uncontrolled Spread*, chapters 10–13; Wright, *The Plague Year*, chapter 12; Borrell, *The First Shots*, chapters 2–4, 7–10, 12–13; and Baker and Glasser, *The Divider*, chapter 23. On the creation of Operation Warp Speed see Mango, *Warp Speed*; Borrell, *The First Shots*, chapters 14–18; and Farrar and Ahuja, *Spike*, chapter 7.

2. See Senate HSGA Majority Staff, *Examination*, 121–123.

3. *PanCAP Adapted: U.S. Government COVID-19 Response Plan*, March 13, 2020 (online), quoting Figure 5, 12.

4. For the President Trump quote see "Trump Says Coronavirus Under Control in the U.S.," *Reuters*, February 24, 2020 (online).

5. Wright, *The Plague Year*, 100–101 (digital).

6. Both quotes can be found in Kathryn Watson, "A Timeline of What Trump Has Said on Coronavirus," *CBS News*, April 3, 2020 (online).

7. "Full control," quoting Olivia Troye in Senate HSGA Majority Staff, *Examination*, 123.

8. Birx, *Silent Invasion*, 54 (digital).

9. Kadlec "off the island" and possible reasons, Senate HSGA Majority Staff, *Examination,* 127.

10. Gaynor in Senate HSGA Majority Staff, *Examination*, 129.

11. Jared Kushner, *Breaking History: A White House Memoir* (New York: Broadside Books, 2022), 368.

12. On Trump, Gaynor, and "surreal" quoting Josh Dozor, Senate HSGA Majority Staff, *Examination*, 130–131. The report includes a photograph of the whiteboard.

13. For other reportage on Azar's status, see, for example, Abutaleb and Paletta, *Nightmare Scenario*, 280 (digital).

14. On OMB's request and Bright, "nickel and diming," Senate HSGA Majority Staff, *Examination*, 139.

15. President Donald J. Trump, Executive Order 13922, "Delegating Authority under the Defense Production Act of 1950 to the Chief Executive Officer of the United States International Development Finance Corporation to Respond to the COVID–19 Outbreak," May 14, 2020.

16. Katherine Eban, "'That's Their Problem': How Jared Kushner Let the Markets Decide America's COVID-19 Fate," *Vanity Fair*, September 17, 2020 (online); "realigned" from *FEMA, Pandemic Response to Coronavirus Disease 2019 (COVID-19): Initial Assessment Report*, January 2021 (online).

17. U.S. House of Representatives Select Subcommittee on the Coronavirus Crisis, "Interview of Scott Atlas," January 7, 2022, 16–17 (online).

18. For Trump and Birx quotes and White House economic staff estimate, see Birx, *Silent Invasion*, 152–163, 193–195 (digital).

19. Wright, *The Plague Year*, 161 (digital).

20. Peter Baker, "George W. Bush Calls for End to Pandemic Partisanship," *New York Times*, May 3, 2020 (online).

21. Meadows quoted in Abutaleb and Paletta, *Nightmare Scenario*, 331.

22. Navarro to Task Force, via Mulvaney and O'Brien, "Request for Immediate Action," February 9, 2020.

23. Bright to Kadlec, "Re: update," February 10, 2020, which, like Navarro's email, is in exhibits 21 and 22 in Bright's May 2020 whistleblower complaint to the Office of the Special Counsel (online).

24. Quotes from a Danzig memo are from Richard Danzig, "A Six Month 'Wartime' Vaccine Program," version 2, March 29, 2020, privately circulated in advance of a March 31 videoconference.

25. For quotes on a "Manhattan Project" for vaccines and drugs see Farrar and Ahuja, *Spike*, 156–158.

26. Susan Athey et al., "In the Race for a Coronavirus Vaccine, We Must Go Big. Really, Really Big." *New York Times,* May 4, 2020 (online).

27. Borrell, *The First Shots*, 169 (digital).

28. Mango, *Warp Speed*, 12 (digital).

29. For quotes by and about President Biden see Ashley Parker et al., "Inside the Successes, Missteps and Failures of Biden's Early Presidency," *Washington Post*, October 22, 2022 (online).

30. For "nearly 2 million a day" see Select Subcommittee on the Coronavirus Crisis, "Interview of Brett Giroir," 52–53. For "junk millions of tests" see Sheri Fink, "Maker of Popular Covid Test Told Factory to Destroy Inventory," *New York Times*, August 20, 2021 (online). On the Biden administration testing push in the winter of 2021–22, see Michael Shear and Sheryl Gay Stolberg, "Biden Promised 500 Million Tests, but Americans Will Have to Wait," *New York Times*, December 22, 2021 (online).

CHAPTER 6. COMMUNITIES IMPROVISE WITH FEW TOOLS

1. For state and local improvisations and innovations, as well as debates about masks see Birx, *Silent Invasion*, chapters 11–15. On stay-at-home orders see Gottlieb, *Uncontrolled Spread*, chapter 11. For data on state opening and closing decisions see "Impact of Opening and Closing Decisions by State," Johns Hopkins University Coronavirus Resource Center, updated September 14, 2022 (online). For N95 mask shortages and procurement see Doug Bock Clark, "Inside the Chaotic, Cutthroat Gray Market for N95 Masks," *New York Times Magazine*, November 17, 2020 (online). On state mask mandates and backlash see Sarah Mervosh et al.,

"Mask Rules Expand across U.S. as Clashes over the Mandates Intensify," *New York Times*, July 16, 2020 (online) and Amy Goldstein, "Anger over Mask Mandates, Other Covid Rules, Spurs States to Curb Power of Public Health Officials," *Washington Post*, December 25, 2021 (online).

For the Jared Kushner quote see Eban, "'That's Their Problem': How Jared Kushner Let the Markets Decide America's COVID-19 Fate." For the Trump quote see Woodward, *The Trump Tapes*, Interview #9.

2. Marcelle Layton quoted in Greg B. Smith, "In Note to Fauci, Top City Doctor Takes Shot at de Blasio's COVID-19 Contact Tracing Program," *City*, January 28, 2021 (online).

3. German Lopez, "Germany Contained Covid-19. Politics Brought It Back." *Vox*, April 21, 2021 (online).

4. Lauren M. Rossen et al., "Excess All-Cause Mortality in the USA and Europe during the COVID-19 Pandemic, 2020 and 2021," *Scientific Reports* 12, no. 1 (November 2022): Table 1 (comparing the period through week 39 of 2020).

5. Tomas Pueyo, "Coronavirus: The Hammer and the Dance,'" *Medium* post, March 19, 2020 (online).

6. For analysis of citizen behavior see Austan Goolsbee and Chad Syverson, "Fear, Lockdown, and Diversion: Comparing Drivers of Pandemic Economic Decline 2020," *Journal of Public Economics* 193 (January 2021): 104311.

7. "Bipartisan Assembly of Governors Support Call to Action to Defeat COVID-19," COVID Collaborative press release, December 10, 2020 (online).

8. Christopher J. Cronin and William N. Evans, "Nursing Home Quality, COVID-19 Deaths, and Excess Mortality," *Journal of Health Economics* 82 (March 2022): 102592; and, for the enormous impact in the first wave of the virus in spring–summer 2020, see CDC reports and Figure 1 in Priya Chidambaran, "Key Questions about the Impact of Coronavirus on Long-Term Care Facilities over Time," *KFF*, September 1, 2020 (online).

9. Sandra Crouse Quinn et al., "Racial Disparities in Exposure, Susceptibility, and Access to Health Care in the US H1N1 Influenza Pandemic," *American Journal of Public Health* 101, no. 2 (February 2011): 285–293.

10. For schools guidance provided by Danielle Allen's team see Danielle Allen et al., "The Path to Zero and Schools: Achieving Pandemic Resilient Teaching and Learning Spaces," July 20, 2020 (online); Danielle Allen et al., "Schools and the Path to Zero: Strategies for Pandemic Resilience in the Face of High Community Spread," December 18, 2020

(online); and Danielle Allen et al., *Roadmap to Healthy Schools: Building Organizational Capacity for Infection Prevention and Control*, Infection Prevention and Control in Schools task force, April 28, 2021 (online).

11. Birx, *Silent Invasion*, 199–201 (digital).

12. Select Subcommittee on the Coronavirus Crisis, "Interview of Brett Giroir," 114–116.

13. "Coronavirus (COVID-19) Update: FDA Continues to Advance Over-the-Counter and Other Screening Test Development," FDA news release, March 31, 2021 (online).

14. Dyani Lewis, "Why the WHO Took Two Years to Say COVID Is Airborne," *Nature*, April 6, 2022 (online).

15. Lea Hamner et al., "High SARS-CoV-2 Attack Rate Following Exposure at a Choir Practice—Skagit County, Washington, March 2020," CDC *Morbidity and Mortality Weekly Report* 69, no. 19 (March 2020): 606–610.

16. Zeynep Tufekci, "Why Did It Take So Long to Accept the Facts about Covid?" *New York Times*, May 7, 2021 (online).

17. For more details on Japanese performance and the Three C's campaign see Dennis Normile, "Japan Ends Its COVID-19 State of Emergency," *Science*, May 26, 2020 (online) and Eric Topol, "The Marked Contrast in Pandemic Outcomes between Japan and the United States," Ground Truths blog, October 8, 2022 (online).

18. Katherine Randall et al., "How Did We Get Here: What Are Droplets and Aerosols and How Far Do They Go? A Historical Perspective on the Transmission of Respiratory Infectious Diseases," *Interface Focus* 11, no. 6 (October 2021): 20210049; and Jose L. Jimenez et al., "What Were the Historical Reasons for the Resistance to Recognizing Airborne Transmission During the COVID-19 Pandemic?," *Indoor Air* 32, no. 8 (August 2022): 13070.

19. See, e.g., Jeremy Howard et al, "An Evidence Review of Face Masks against Covid-19," *Proceedings of the National Academy of Sciences*, January 26, 2021 (online); Tori Cowger et al., "Lifting Universal Masking in Schools—Covid-19 Incidence among Students and Staff," *New England Journal of Medicine*, November 9, 2022 (online).

20. For a timeline of mask guidance see Marie Fazio, "How Mask Guidelines Have Evolved," *New York Times*, April 27, 2021 (online).

21. For ASPR procurement efforts and Project Airbridge see Congressional Research Service, *COVID-19 and Domestic PPE Production and Distribution: Issues and Policy Options*, December 7, 2020 (online).

22. Baker and Glasser, *The Divider*, chapter 23; Wright, *The Plague Year*, 159 (digital).

23. Associated Press, "Trump on Mask Wearing: 'I Don't Think' I'll Do It," *New York Times* (video), April 3, 2020 (online).

24. Abutaleb and Paletta, *Nightmare Scenario*, 335–336 (digital).

25. Asa Hutchinson, "Gov. Asa Hutchinson: to Fight Coronavirus Wear a Mask—New Survey Shows Most Americans Agree," *Fox News*, August 22, 2020 (online).

26. For Georgia example see Meagan Flynn and Marisa Iati, "Georgia Gov. Brian Kemp Sues Atlanta over Mask Requirement as Coronavirus Surges in the State," *Washington Post*, July 16, 2020 (online); for Wisconsin example see Todd Richmond, "Wisconsin Mask Mandate Struck Down by State Supreme Court," *Chicago Tribune*, March 31, 2021 (online); for North Dakota example see Jeremy Turley, "North Dakota Bans State Officials from Mandating Masks Despite Gov. Doug Burgum Veto," *Dickinson Press*, April 22, 2021 (online).

27. Rossen et al., "Excess All-Cause Mortality in the USA and Europe," Table 1 (comparing the period from week 40 of 2020 through the first half of 2021).

28. UNESCO Institute for Statistics, "Global Monitoring of School Closures Caused by COVID-19," March 2022 (online).

29. Cassandra Willyard, "COVID and Schools: The Evidence for Reopening Safely," *Nature*, July 7, 2021 (online).

30. For details on the learning losses and other effects of disrupted schooling see Cory Turner, "6 Things We've Learned about How the Pandemic Disrupted Learning," *NPR*, June 22, 2022 (online).

31. For details on the San Antonio school testing program see Brooke Crum, "San Antonio School District to Roll Out Free COVID-19 Testing for All Teachers and Students," *San Antonio Report*, January 5, 2021 (online), and Emily Anthes and Sabrina Imbler, "'I Need an Army': Across America, Schools Cram for Their Covid Tests," *New York Times*, September 25, 2021 (online).

32. For details on the Massachusetts school testing program see Calley Jones, "Broad Institute Is Processing Pooled COVID-19 Tests for Massachusetts K-12 Schools," Broad Institute news release, February 25, 2021 (online) and Jesse S. Boehm, "The Power of Parent Scientists," *Cell* 184, no. 9 (April 2021): 2263–2270.

33. For the school reopening road map produced by Danielle Allen's group, working with the Covid Collaborative, Brown University's School

of Public Health and the New America Foundation, see Danielle Allen et al., *Roadmap to Healthy Schools: Building Organizational Capacity for Infection Prevention and Control*, Infection Prevention and Control in Schools Task Force, April 28, 2021 (online).

34. Jeneen Interlandi, "Can the C.D.C. Be Fixed?" *New York Times Magazine*, June 16, 2021 (online).

35. For 2021–22 school guidance see "U.S. Department of Education Releases 'Return to School Roadmap' to Support Students, Schools, Educators, and Communities in Preparing for the 2021–2022 School Year," U.S. Department of Education press release, August 2, 2021 (online) and the White House, "Memorandum on Ensuring a Safe Return to In-Person School for the Nation's Children," August 18, 2021 (online).

36. U.S. Department of Education, National Center for Education Progress, National Assessment of Educational Progress (NAEP), 2022 Mathematics and Reading Report Card. On women returning to the workforce, Stephanie Ferguson and Isabella Lucy, "Data Deep Dive: A Decline of Women in the Workforce," U.S. Chamber of Commerce, April 27, 2022 (online).

37. See, for example, L. Radhakrishnan, R.T. Leeb, R.H. Bitsko, et al, "Pediatric Emergency Department Visits Associated with Mental Health Conditions Before and During the COVID-19 Pandemic—United States, January 2019–January 2022," *MMWR Morbidity & Mortality Weekly Report*, vol. 71: 319–324 (2022) (online).

CHAPTER 7. THE HEALTHCARE SYSTEM FRAYS

1. For proposals to strengthen the ability of the healthcare systems to prepare for and respond to crises see Disaster Preparedness & Response Initiative, *National Dialogue for Healthcare Innovation: Framework for Private-Public Collaboration on Disaster Preparedness and Response*, February 2021 (online). To see how leaders saw the medical supply issues before the Covid war, see the summary of the National Academies workshop, *Medical Product Shortages During Disasters: Opportunities to Predict, Prevent, and Respond* (2018) (online). For personal stories and insight into the experience of frontline healthcare works during the Covid crisis see the podcast series *The Nocturnists*.

For "thirty-six hundred died" see Jane Spencer, *Guardian*, Christina Jewett, "12 Months of Trauma: More Than 3,600 US Health Workers Died in Covid's First Year," *Kaiser Health News*, April 8, 2021 (online).

2. For more on Lloyd Armbrust see Tom Simonite, "Covid Forced America to Make More Stuff. What Happens Now?" *Wired*, May 17, 2021 (online).

3. The 60 percent figure and quote by Bryan Sexton from Oliver Whang, "Physician Burnout Has Reached Distressing Levels, New Research Finds," *New York Times*, September 29, 2022 (online).

4. For "one in five healthcare workers" see Gaby Galvin, "Nearly 1 in 5 Health Care Workers Have Quit Their Jobs During the Pandemic," *Morning Consult*, October 4, 2021 (online). On ID training, Pien Huang, "Newest Doctors Shun Infectious Diseases Specialty," *Shots: Health News from NPR*, December 12, 2022 (online).

CHAPTER 8. TRUST AND CONFIDENCE BREAK DOWN

1. For a study of false news online see Soroush Vosoughi, Deb Roy, and Sinan Aral, "The Spread of True and False News Online," *Science* 359, no. 6380 (March 2018): 1146–1151. For strategies on combating misinformation and disinformation see Tara Kirk Sell et al., *National Priorities to Combat Misinformation and Disinformation for COVID-19 and Future Public Health Threats: A Call for a National Strategy*, Johns Hopkins Center for Health Security, March 2021 (online). For background on the Tuskegee study see Vann R. Newkirk II, "A Generation of Bad Blood," *Atlantic*, June 17, 2016 (online).

2. National Academies of Sciences, Engineering, and Medicine, *Building Communication Capacity to Counter Infectious Disease Threats: Proceedings of a Workshop* (Washington, DC: National Academies Press, 2017).

3. Baruch Fischhoff, "Making Decisions in a COVID-19 World," *JAMA* 324, no. 2 (June 2020): 139-140.

4. National Academies of Sciences, Engineering, and Medicine, *Framework for Equitable Allocation of COVID-19 Vaccine* (Washington, DC: National Academies Press, 2020).

5. Baruch Fischhoff, "The COVID Communication Breakdown," *Foreign Affairs*, October 4, 2021 (online).

6. Statistics on removed and labeled posts from Guy Rosen, "Moving Past the Finger Pointing," Meta (formerly Facebook) company press release, July 17, 2021 (online). For unvaccinated hospitalized patients see Aaron Blake, "Yes, It's Still a Pandemic of the Unvaccinated—Arguably Even More So Now," *Washington Post*, February 3, 2022 (online).

7. Baruch Fischhoff, "The Sciences of Science Communication," *Proceedings of the National Academy of Sciences* 110 (August 2013): 14033-14039.

8. On West Virginia's communication approach, see Laura Strickler and Lisa Cavazuti, "'We Crushed It': How Did West Virginia Become a National Leader in Covid Vaccination?" *NBC News*, January 31, 2021 (online); "Data-driven Communication about COVID-19 Vaccines in West Virginia," Centers for Disease Control and Prevention community feature, September 30, 2021 (online); "West Virginia COVID-19 Vaccines Communication Toolkit Version 4," State of West Virginia, January 18, 2021 (online).

9. "Rural Americans Share Personal Stories to Inspire Confidence in COVID-19 Vaccines in Local Communities and Nationwide," Covid Collaborative press release, October 19, 2021 (online).

10. For American Indian communities see Raymond Foxworth et al., "Covid-19 Vaccination in American Indians and Alaska Natives—Lessons from Effective Community Responses," *New England Journal of Medicine* 385, no. 26 (December 2021): 2403–2406.

11. "The Ad Council and COVID Collaborative Reveal 'It's Up to You' Campaigns to Educate Millions of Americans about COVID-19 Vaccines," Covid Collaborative press release, February 25, 2021 (online).

12. The White House, *National Strategy for the COVID-19 Response and Pandemic Preparedness*, January 2021 (online).

13. Cary Funk and Alec Tyson, "Intent to Get a COVID-19 Vaccine Rises to 60% as Confidence in Research and Development Process Increases," *Pew Research Center*, December 3, 2020 (online).

14. Adam Liptak, "Supreme Court Blocks Biden's Virus Mandate for Large Employers," *New York Times*, January 13, 2022 (online).

15. Donald Trump vaccine quotes from Baker and Glasser, *Divider*, 643–644.

16. Lunna Lopes et al., "KFF COVID-19 Vaccine Monitor: July 2022," KFF, July 26, 2022, Figure 13.

17. David Leonhardt, "A Public Health Success Story," *New York Times*, October 4, 2022 (online).

18. Rossen et al., "Excess All-Cause Mortality in the USA and Europe," Table 1 (comparing the period from week 27 of 2021 through the rest of the year); see also David Wallace-Wells, "What a Single Metric Tells Us about the Pandemic," *New York*, March 26, 2022 (online).

19. Range of excess deaths in 2021–22 estimated in Alyssa Bilinski, Kathryn Thompson, and Ezekiel J. Emanuel, "COVID-19 and Excess All-

Cause Mortality in the US and 20 Comparison Countries, June 2021–March 2022," *JAMA Network Research Letter*, November 18, 2022 (online).

20. Arnav Shah et al., "How Can the U.S. Catch Up with Other Countries on COVID-19 Vaccination?" Commonwealth Fund blog post, December 15, 2021 (online) and "See How Vaccinations Are Going in Your County and State," *New York Times* data tracker, updated October 20, 2022 (online).

CHAPTER 9. FIGHTING BACK WITH DRUGS AND VACCINES

1. On building a biopharma industrial base see the MITRE Corporation, *Building a Sustainable Biopreparedness Industrial Base*, March 2022 (online) and Kendall Hoyt et al., *MCMx: A Proposal for a Federal Authority to Enhance Speed, Scale and Access to Medical Countermeasures*, Harvard Medical School Program in Global Public Policy and Social Change Task Force on Medical Countermeasures, May 28, 2021 (online). For vaccine financing see Jonathan T. Vu et al., "Financing Vaccines for Global Health Security," *Journal of Investment Management* 20, no. 2 (2022): 51–67. For background on mRNA as a vaccine platform see Jeffrey B. Ulmer et al., "Vaccines 'on demand': Science Fiction or a Future Reality," *Expert Opinion on Drug Discovery* 10, no. 2 (January 2015): 101-106. For the development of COVID-19 therapeutics see Dan Werb, *The Invisible Siege: The Rise of Coronaviruses and the Search for a Cure* (New York: Crown, digital ed. 2022), chapters 7–16; Gottlieb, *Uncontrolled Spread*, chapter 16; and Quammen, *Breathless*, chapter 53. On COVID-19 vaccine design see Borrell, *The First Shots*, chapters 1, 5–6, 11; Quammen, *Breathless*, chapters 54–58; Gottlieb, *Uncontrolled Spread*, chapter 17; Werb, *The Invisible Siege*, chapters 7–16; and Gina Kolata and Benjamin Mueller, "Halting Progress and Happy Accidents: How mRNA Vaccines Were Made," *New York Times*, January 15, 2022 (online). On Operation Warp Speed in action see Mango, *Warp Speed* and Borrell, *The First Shots*, chapters 16–27.

For development of an Ebola vaccine see Helen Branswell, "'Against All Odds': The Inside Story of How Scientists across Three Continents Produced an Ebola Vaccine," *Stat*, January 7, 2020 (online).

2. For the British technical report see U.K. Department of Health and Social Care, *Technical Report on the COVID-19 Pandemic in the UK*, December 2022 (online).

3. "Low-cost Dexamethasone Reduces Death by Up to One-third in Hospitalised Patients with Severe Respiratory Complications of COVID-19," Statement from the Chief Investigators of the Randomised Evaluation of COVID-19 Therapy (RECOVERY) Trial, June 16, 2020 (online).

4. See, for example, H. Clifford Lane and Anthony Fauci, "Research in the Context of a Pandemic," *New England Journal of Medicine*, February 25, 2021 (online).

5. See Charles Piller, "Former FDA Leaders Decry Emergency Authorization of Malaria Drugs for Coronavirus," *Science*, April 8, 2020 (online).

6. When asked about this episode, Marks told us that the therapy had to be paired with an assay to determine that the plasma would be effective. This associated requirement, he said, was not followed.

7. Philip Krause, et al, "Considerations in boosting COVID-19 Vaccine Immune Responses," *Lancet*, September 13, 2021 (online).

8. Jeffrey Shuren and Timothy Stenzel, "South Korea's Implementation of a COVID-19 National Testing Strategy," *Health Affairs*, May 25, 2021 (online).

9. For Emergent BioSolutions see Sharon LaFraniere et al., "The F.D.A. Tells Johnson & Johnson That about 60 Million Doses Made at a Troubled Plant Cannot Be Used," *New York Times*, June 11, 2021 (online). For cancellation of Emergent's contract see Andrew Jeong, "U.S. Cancels Multimillion-Dollar Deal with Coronavirus Vaccine Maker Whose Plant Ruined Johnson & Johnson Doses," *Washington Post*, November 5, 2021 (online).

10. Details and quotes from MITRE's 2019 report on BARDA provided by a former Trump administration official.

11. For some details on President Trump's illness and treatment see Werb, *The Invisible Siege*, chapter 14 and Gottlieb, *Uncontrolled Spread*, chapter 16.

12. Arman Shafiee, et al., "Ivermectin under Scrutiny: A Systematic Review and Meta-Analysis of Efficacy and Possible Sources of Controversies in COVID-19 Patients," *Virology Journal* 19, no. 1 (June 2022): 102.

13. Carl Zimmer, "New Covid Pills Offer Hope as Omicron Looms," *New York Times*, December 7, 2021 (online).

14. Mango, *Warp Speed*, 12 (digital).

15. Arthur Allen, "How Pfizer Won the Pandemic, Reaping Outsize Profit and Influence," *Kaiser Health News*, July 5, 2022 (online).

16. Executive Office of the President, Letter from President's Council of Advisors on Science and Technology to President Barack Obama, November 2016 (online).

17. Rachel Cohrs, "The Trump Administration Quietly Spent Billions in Hospital Funds on Operation Warp Speed," *Stat*, March 2, 2021 (online).

18. Quotes from Bill LaPlante in Valerie Insinna, "Multi-year Procurement for Munitions Would Help Stabilize Industry: LaPlante," *Breaking Defense*, September 7, 2022 (online).

CHAPTER 10. STRATEGY FOR A GLOBAL WAR

1. On the global vaccine efforts and COVAX see Farrar and Ahuja, *Spike*, chapters 7–8; Jillian Deutsch and Sarah Wheaton, "How Europe Fell behind on Vaccines," *Politico*, January 27, 2021 (online); Seth Berkley, "COVAX Explained," Gavi, the Vaccine Alliance explainer post, September 3, 2020 (online); Benjamin Mueller and Rebecca Robbins, "Where a Vast Global Vaccination Program Went Wrong," *New York Times*, August 2, 2021 (online). For background on CEPI's hundred-day vaccine goal see Coalition for Epidemic Preparedness Innovations, *Delivering Pandemic Vaccines in 100 Days*, September 2022 (online). On calls for U.S. leadership in global vaccination efforts see Stephen Morrison et al., *The Time Is Now for U.S. Global Leadership on Covid-19 Vaccines*, CSIS Commission on Strengthening America's Health Security, April 2021 (online).

For Zhang Yongzhen see Jon Cohen, "Chinese Researchers Reveal Draft Genome of Virus Implicated in Wuhan Pneumonia Outbreak," *Science*, January 11, 2020 (online).

2. Gavi, *2021 Annual Progress Report*, September 29, 2022 (online).

3. Figures for vaccine candidate success rates from Berkley, "COVAX Explained."

4. Matina Stevis-Gridneff and Lara Jakes, "World Leaders Join to Pledge $8 Billion for Vaccine as U.S. Goes It Alone," *New York Times*, May 4, 2020 (online).

5. "France, Germany, Italy and the Netherlands Working Together to Find a Vaccine for Countries in Europe and Beyond," news release from the government of the Netherlands, June 3, 2020 (online).

6. Olivia Goldhill, "We Have Enough Covid Vaccines for Most of the World. But Rich Countries Are Stockpiling More Than They Need for Boosters." *Stat*, December 13, 2021 (online).

7. This argument is developed in, for example, Richard Danzig, "Vaccines as Instruments for National Security," *The Bridge* [National Academy of Engineering], December 15, 2020 (online).

8. As of November 4, 2022, COVAX had delivered 1.83 billion Covid vaccine doses to 146 countries according to "Factbox: Vaccines Delivered under COVAX Sharing Scheme for Poorer Countries," *Reuters*, November 4, 2022 (online).

9. Thomas J. Bollyky et al., "Global Vaccination Must Be Swifter," *Nature*, March 28, 2022 (online). For a critical report on the ACT-Accelerator that echoes these points, see the summary and links in Ann Danaiya Usher, "ACT-A: 'The international architecture did not work for us'," *Lancet*, October 20, 2022 (online).

10. Chad P. Bown, "COVID-19 Vaccine Supply Chains and the Defense Production Act," Peterson Institute for International Economics working paper, June 2022, 17 (online).

11. Bown, "COVID-19 Vaccine Supply Chains and the Defense Production Act," 17.

12. Bown, "COVID-19 Vaccine Supply Chains and the Defense Production Act," 19.

CHAPTER 11. AMERICA THE COMPETENT?

1. Niall Ferguson, *Doom: The Politics of Catastrophe* (New York: Penguin Press, 2021), 383.

2. CEPI, *Delivering Pandemic Vaccines in 100 Days*, 5.

3. Analogy to Formula 1 racing in CEPI, *Delivering Pandemic Vaccines in 100 Days*, 24.

4. On control strategies see Andreas Handel, Ira Longini Jr., and Rustom Antia, "What Is the Best Control Strategy for Multiple Infectious Disease Outbreaks?," *Proc. Biol. Sci.*, 2007 (online).

5. Stephen Platt, *Imperial Twilight: The Opium War and the End of China's Last Golden Age* (New York: Knopf, 2018), 233 (following the work of William Rowe).

INDEX

for marginalized communities, 58
struggle from lack of demand for, 196
condition, Kingdon on problem
compared to, 25, 306n27
"Conditions of Participation" of CMS,
for hospital preparedness, 189
contact tracing approach, 146–147
contagion
of SARS-CoV-1 lesser, 5
in schools and community spread, 180
containment failures, 81, 117–119
biomedical surveillance absence,
102–107
first warnings, 82–87
influenza pandemic of 1918 and, 87–95
literature on, 311n1
testing problems, 107–113
influenza pandemic of 1918 and, 87–95
containment policy designs
CDC travel screening, 97, 101
Germany success in, 98–99
mobilization neglect, 97, 117
Obama "playbook" and, 95–96
screening system and testing, 97–98
South Korea success in, 98–99
U.S. software absence, 100–101
convalescent blood plasma treatment,
inefficiency of, 227–228
Corbett, Kizzmekia, 245
Coronavirus Aid, Relief, and Economic
Security (CARES) Act, 122–123
Coronavirus Infectious Disease–2019
(COVID-19)
description of, 4–5
influenza 1918–1919 compared to, 4,
13–14, 302nn1–2
SARS-CoV-2 cause of, 4–5
two early case lineages identified for,
33
two spillover events for, 32
costs, of Covid-19, 10–12
Council of State and Territorial
Epidemiologists report, 59–60
COVAX. See COVID-19 Vaccines
Global Access

Covid Collaborative, 274
consortium effort and, 24, 154,
212–213
vaccination education campaign, 215
Covid commission, U.S. neglect to
create, 1, 24
COVID Data Tracker, of CDC, on
hospitalization numbers, 9, 303n6
Covid Tracking Project, at Johns
Hopkins University, 105
Covid-19. See Coronavirus Infectious
Disease-2019
Covid-19 IFRs, influenza of 1918
compared to, 4, 302n2
COVID-19 Vaccines Global Access
(COVAX), 263, 263 (fig.)
clinical trials, 266
funding difficulties, 265
low-income country vaccination from,
269–270
vaccine candidates of, 264–265
vaccine development of, 264
vaccine nationalism causing delays
for, 270
world vaccine procurement entity, 14
COVID-NET, 104, 314n22
Crimson Contagion, 115–117, 222, 314n1
Crisis Standard of Care (CSC) hospital
plans, 195–196
cultures, of governance, 17–20

Danzig, Richard, 134–136, 261–262,
316n24
DARPA. See Defense Advanced Research
Projects Agency
data exchange
Council of State and Territorial
Epidemiologists on challenges to,
59–60
healthcare system necessary, 198
from states to CDC, 62–63
Defense Advanced Research Projects
Agency (DARPA)
Giroir management role of, 64–65
Moderna support from, 245, 248, 253

public problem-solving in, 20–21
surgical toolkits tools, 158 (fig.)
polio vaccinations, during 1950s, 55
political challenge, 22, 24, 25, 26. *See also*
Democrats; Republicans
political polarization, from Trump,
207–209
political system, Wuhan Institute of
Virology and, 39
polymerase chain reaction (PCR) tests,
107–108, 166–168
Pottinger, Matt
China physician phone call to, 87–88
on China travel ban to U.S., 88–89
as deputy national security adviser,
87, 89 (photo)
NSC role in Coronavirus Task Force,
117
response involvement decline, 121
at Trump PDB, 88, 313n11
White House and NSC memos,
132–133
PPE. *See* personal protective equipment
pre-healthcare data streams monitoring,
41
premature death figures
global, 8, 303n5
U.S., 8, 23, 303n5
The Premonition (Lewis), 16
President's Daily Brief (PDB), Pottinger
on crisis at Trump, 88, 313n11
Prestige Ameritech, as N95 masks
manufacturer, 85–86
prevention, situation awareness
improvement for, 27–28, 40–47
prevention and warning challenge, in
global war, 5, 27–28
Prior Preparation Prevents Poor
Performance (five P's), of Baker,
101
private healthcare system, government
bailout for, 22
problem, Kingdon on condition
compared to, 25, 306n27
problem-solving software, 20–22

Project Airbridge, of Kushner, 125–126,
175, 191
Project BioShield, underfunding of, 237
proning technique, 200–201
protease inhibitors, of Pfizer Paxlovid,
239–240, 242–243, 276
protein subunit vaccine, 246
Novavax and, 248, 249, 263 (fig.), 275
Sanofi-GSK and, 249, 263 (fig.)
public health community
of CDC and health departments, 68
CDC leadership of, 76
healthcare systems connection with,
72
The Public Health Crisis Survival Guide
(Sharfstein), 81
public health data, Redfield on lack of
system for, 62–63
Public Health Emergency Fund, less
than $60,000 when Covid hit, 78
Public Health Emergency Medical
Countermeasures Enterprise
(PHEMCE), 74, 75
Public Health Emergency Preparedness
(PHEP) program, federal funding
through, 60–61
public health professions, literature on,
309n1
Public Health Service
of Cleveland, 53
Commissioned Corps of, 78
Giroir of, 63–64
public health system
challenges to, 22
core capabilities neglect, 59–61
funding and qualified people absence
in, 60
healthcare system disconnect by,
58–59, 71
layered jurisdictional authority in,
56–57
limited reforms for, 23
positive health from, 204
U.S. lack of community health
workers in, 57–58

PublicAffairs is a publishing house founded in 1997. It is a tribute to the standards, values, and flair of three persons who have served as mentors to countless reporters, writers, editors, and book people of all kinds, including me.

I. F. STONE, proprietor of *I. F. Stone's Weekly*, combined a commitment to the First Amendment with entrepreneurial zeal and reporting skill and became one of the great independent journalists in American history. At the age of eighty, Izzy published *The Trial of Socrates*, which was a national bestseller. He wrote the book after he taught himself ancient Greek.

BENJAMIN C. BRADLEE was for nearly thirty years the charismatic editorial leader of *The Washington Post*. It was Ben who gave the *Post* the range and courage to pursue such historic issues as Watergate. He supported his reporters with a tenacity that made them fearless and it is no accident that so many became authors of influential, best-selling books.

ROBERT L. BERNSTEIN, the chief executive of Random House for more than a quarter century, guided one of the nation's premier publishing houses. Bob was personally responsible for many books of political dissent and argument that challenged tyranny around the globe. He is also the founder and longtime chair of Human Rights Watch, one of the most respected human rights organizations in the world.

•   •   •

For fifty years, the banner of Public Affairs Press was carried by its owner Morris B. Schnapper, who published Gandhi, Nasser, Toynbee, Truman, and about 1,500 other authors. In 1983, Schnapper was described by *The Washington Post* as "a redoubtable gadfly." His legacy will endure in the books to come.

Peter Osnos, *Founder*